Praise for

the water secret

"As someone who has used Dr. Murad's products for years, I love what they've done for my skin. With *The Water Secret*, Dr. Murad shows us that topical skin care is just one piece of the puzzle."
—Joy Behar, Emmy® Award winner, co-host of *The View* and host of *The Joy Behar Show*

"The principles in *The Water Secret* will transform your health inside and out. I started seeing Dr. Murad because of all the damage I'd done to my skin as a result of shooting *Survivor*. With his Inclusive approach, he not only helped me reverse a lot of the damage, he's shown me how to optimize my health on a daily basis."
—Jeff Probst, Emmy® Award winner, host of *Survivor*

"Dr. Murad translates his insights into health and the science of the aging process into a practical plan for building a better, more beautiful life. Anyone can live inclusively and everyone should!"
—Debbie Gibson, singer/songwriter

"Dr. Murad is a true innovator. In *The Water Secret*, he clearly demonstrates how, through his Inclusive Health approach, you will not only *look* your best, but *be* your best . . . at any age!"
—Josie Bissett, actress, *The Secret Life of the American Teenager* and *Melrose Place*

"A groundbreaking theory about how to look and feel—and be—younger from one of the country's leading dermatologists. Could this be the fountain of youth?"
—Valerie Latona, editor-in-chief, *Shape* magazine

"*The Water Secret* outlines a pragmatic, easy-to-follow health regimen highlighting the scientific reasons it works—making it simple for everyone to achieve optimal beauty from the inside out."
—Elaine D'Farley, beauty director, *Self* magazine

"If you want to look prettier, feel happier, and be healthier, buy this book!"
—Jean Godfrey-June, beauty director, *Lucky* magazine

"Dr. Murad's research in The Science of Cellular Water™ may prove to be the breakthrough we've been looking for."
—William V. R. Shellow, M. D., Clinical Professor of Medicine (Dermatology), UCLA

the water secret

THE CELLULAR BREAKTHROUGH TO LOOK AND FEEL 10 YEARS YOUNGER

Dr. Howard Murad, M.D.

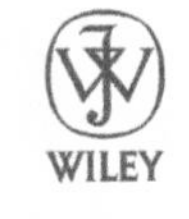

John Wiley & Sons, Inc.

Published by John Wiley & Sons, Inc., Hoboken, New Jersey

Design by Forty-Five Degree Design LLC

Library of Congress Cataloging-in-Publication Data:

Murad, Howard.
 The water secret : the cellular breakthrough to look and feel ten years younger / Howard Murad.
 p. cm.
 Includes index.
 ISBN 978-0-470-55470-8 (pbk.); ISBN 978-0-470-63495-0 (ebk); ISBN 978-0-470-63496-7 (ebk); ISBN 978-0-470-63497-4 (ebk)
 1. Hydrotherapy. 2. Aging—Prevention. 3. Skin—Care and hygiene. 4. Beauty, Personal. I. Title.
 RM811.M965 2010
 615.8'53—dc22

2010006500

Printed in the United States of America

10 9 8 7 6 5 4 3 2

Contents

Introduction	One Doctor's Crusade to Find the Secret to Optimal Health	1
1	How Well Are You, *Really*?	13
2	Three Kinds of Aging and a Three-Pronged Approach to Care	35
3	Eat Your Water, Don't Drink It	57
4	Ten Simple Steps to Living by the Water Secret: Meal Plans and Recipes	87
5	It's Not What You Eat, It's What You *Don't* Eat	131
6	What the Fittest People Know That You Don't	159
7	Why Skin Care Is Health Care	179
8	Combat Cultural Stress	211
Epilogue	Your Best Is Yet to Come	249
	Acknowledgments	257
	Index	261

INTRODUCTION

One Doctor's Crusade to Find the Secret to Optimal Health

True health is not the absence of disease.
True health is emotional, physical,
mental, and spiritual well-being.

What I am about to share with you has been in the making for more than thirty years, and will single-handedly change the way you think about living your life. Based on the untold story of aging, this message and set of strategies have the potential to radically enhance the quality of your health, your looks, and just about everything that makes you, well, *you*.

What I have discovered and proven through treating thousands of patients since my initial experiments with the Water Secret is that *the key to vibrant health from the inside out lies in maintaining strong cells that can retain water the way younger cells do*. It's as simple as that. If you can repair your cells' membranes (from brain cells and heart cells to connective tissue and your outermost skin cells that present you to the world) while attracting water and nutrients to them, you can fight aging and disease. You can help your body heal and rejuvenate itself so you not only look fantastic, but you also feel healthier, revitalized, and ready to participate in life to the fullest. And the best part of this program is that you can start from anywhere, no matter how fast you think your age clock has been ticking for whatever reason. The Water Secret is for everyone regardless of age, health, and habits. I'm here to prove that you can take charge of your personal remote control today and flip to a different channel, where you'll greet a younger, invigorated new self in as little as ten weeks. This is the time it takes for virtually every cell in your body to replenish itself; so, in a lot of ways, you can really be a whole "new" person within ten weeks.

Before I explain why water—and in particular *cellular* water—is so important, let me ask one question: on a scale of 1 to 10, how well are you, for real? We all get the "How are you?" on a regular basis from friends and acquaintances, to which many of us reply reflexively, "I'm pretty good" or "I'm fine. How are *you*?" And so the fibbing goes. But if you were to stop and really think about your well-being—how you are physically and emotionally—could you truthfully answer "*Terrific, fabulous, better than ever*"? Would you give yourself an impressive 10? Would someone you don't know peg you at five to ten years younger than your chronological age?

In truth, very few people can honestly say that they feel their absolute best and look it, too. In my experience, most people put themselves at a 7 or maybe an 8. Even those who believe they lead healthy, robust lives give themselves a 9 and believe they (like anyone else) have room for improvement.

This book is going to show you how to move toward—and hopefully achieve—that perfect 10 and take as many as ten years off your physical age. No gimmicks; no needles; no surgery or pharmaceuticals required. In fact, you can take a short test in the first chapter that will help you to know how well you really are right now and where you could potentially be in the near future. Accomplishing this is easier than you think. You will not have to train for a marathon, go low-carb, force-feed yourself a food that you can't stand no matter how it's cooked, pick up an expensive habit that you hate, or commence a program during which you count down the days till it's over. Much to the contrary, you will merely make slight shifts in what you already do, proceed at your own pace, and learn a way of living that's sustainable *for you*. I've designed this book to be highly accessible and practical for every type of person in the hopes that you keep this on your shelf as a reference for years to come.

You'll be amazed at the transformation you can make through small *additions* to your diet alongside a few simple strategies for nourishing your skin and your emotional well-being. Three components—internal, topical, and emotional self-care—encompass my formula for Inclusive Health care that helps protect and promote the integrity of your cells to keep your body as "young" as possible. At the heart of the last component (emotional self-care) is the ability to manage a new category of stress that runs amok these days and does more damage to us than we realize. As you will learn in this book, Cultural Stress is proving to be the sneakiest silent killer of all. It's what you experience as you merge onto a congested highway with thoughts of being late again and not having time to check your e-mails before 9:00 A.M. or to respond to the twenty messages marked high-priority(!) from yesterday. (And despite your hyperconnections to others through modern technology, a part of you feels lonely and isolated.)

This pervasive scenario has nothing to do with "survival of the fittest." Cultural Stress is wearing and tearing us down daily in ways we never thought possible—so much so that I've commenced my own studies and offered grants to researchers to explore the impact of Cultural Stress. You'll be among the first to read some of the astonishing new evidence. Are there solutions to combating this new stress? Certainly. In some regards, this book is all about doing *less* while accomplishing more. Sounds like a tall order, but it won't seem that way once you experience the Water Secret working within your body.

So if you have been frustrated or unhappy with how you feel and look, despite personal health challenges or conditions, then you've come to the right place. Chances are, you picked up this book for a reason. Maybe it's the chronic exhaustion, the lack of a healthy glow, the thinning hair, the brittle nails, or the extra ten pounds you didn't have a year ago. Maybe it's the "older" person looking back at you in the mirror, a recent diagnosis from your doctor, or simply the fear of getting sick and watching your life hit an abysmal ditch. Or maybe you're among those lucky few who are in excellent health but you want to do more and learn a fresh approach to preserving your health and longevity. I'm going to present a revolutionary way to think about taking care of yourself based on the most essential ingredient to life second only to oxygen: water. As you'll soon find out, water is our best life preserver.

My Journey

I was seven years old when I arrived in the United States from Baghdad with my multigenerational family of eight. We lived in a six-hundred-square-foot apartment in New York City during those early years. With a father who had instilled in me the value of hard work and an education, I was the prototypical dedicated student and a curious learner—eager to make a profound contribution to the world and have a role in the lives of others. Never in my wildest dreams could I have predicted, though, that I'd be part of the transformation of skin care as we know it, and ultimately, of health care.

Unfortunately, we live in a world where health care is administered mostly à la carte and focused primarily on treatment rather than prevention. If you have a nagging cold, you visit an internist. If you have heart palpitations, you see a cardiologist. If you have arthritis, you find a rheumatologist. If you have a skin tag or an incessant rash, you see a dermatologist. But what happens when you just don't as feel as well as you'd like and none of these doctors has a straightforward answer? How can you take charge of your health by addressing your cells' most basic need—water—and repair cells as they age so they continue to function at their best, rather than waiting to treat a specific ailment once those cells have lost their optimal functionality?

Therein lies the promise of the Water Secret, a new way of looking at health that embraces a multipronged—*inclusive*—approach to slowing aging down and in some cases totally reversing the process by honoring a cell's most fundamental need. It won't just make your heart stronger, your aches lessen, and your skin clearer; it also has the potential to radically enhance the condition of your overall health so you stand a greater chance of escaping common diseases that afflict millions. The Water Secret honors proven strategies in both ancient and modern medicine that fortify the body with the tools to function optimally. My hope is that more and more medical doctors combine ancient medicine with modern science to treat everything from colds to cancer.

I attribute my appreciation for teamwork and multidisciplinary approaches to problem-solving to my days in Vietnam. When I came home and pursued dermatology, I was eager to set the bar on patient care and approach the practice with an appreciation for all areas of medicine. During my early years in private practice, though, I was struck by the number of patients who were not getting the help they needed from established treatment protocols. I looked for innovative ways to help my patients, taking advantage of my background as a pharmacist to create my first acne and antiaging formulas. Back then, there were very few effective products available to address things such as acne, wrinkles, age spots, and pigmentation.

So it was out of this incredible need to fill this void that in the 1980s I became one of the major innovators in cosmeceutical as well as nutraceutical research. I began to prescribe supplements and compounded formulas specifically for each patient. In 1989 I founded the Murad Skin Research Laboratory and developed the first "Dr. Brand." By then I had treated nearly ten thousand patients with my personally blended formulas and thus began my journey that would completely change the skin care field as a whole, as well as dermatology as it is practiced today. Upgraded, sophisticated descendants of my initial products are still widely popular.

Eager to expand my ability to help people have healthier skin, I began to make my professional products available to doctors' offices and salons and to provide educational support to ensure that they could be used safely to maximum effect.

The gap between cold cream—which defined the state of the art for aestheticians at the time—and the prescription skin treatments available to doctors was huge. I made it a mission of mine to successfully bridge that gap one formula at a time, starting with my first alpha-hydroxy acid (AHA) products for professionals. I also made it a mission to transform the spa industry by encouraging aestheticians to train with dermatologists to achieve the highest standards in professional treatments as well as to promote overall wellness in their clients. Today not only have the terms "aesthetician" and "cosmeceutical" become part of our common vernacular, but also you see alpha-hydroxy acids in thousands of beauty products to help exfoliate and revitalize skin. You can imagine how crazy it first sounded to use an "acid" on skin! When I initially began speaking with aestheticians at trade shows, there was considerable resistance, but now AHAs are a normal part of a skin health and beauty regimen.

Continually searching for new and better ways to help people reach their skin health goals, in 1995 I began to encourage my patients to stop neglecting the 80 percent of our skin that topical products can't reach. In doing so, I developed a revolutionary inside-out approach to skin care that incorporates dietary supplements to improve the health and appearance of skin by improving the strength of each cell in the body. To treat the skin as an isolated component of the body is like using a small brush to touch up the outdoor paint on a house rocked off its foundation and about to crumble under years of neglect and disrepair. My new way of looking at treatment earned me recognition as a founding father of internal skin care. It also opened the door for me to discover the Water Secret.

In 2007 I opened the new Murad Inclusive Health Spa in Los Angeles, a diagnostic and medical spa completely based on the Water Secret. This multimillion-dollar facility incorporates healing and medical philosophies from all over the world—Western and Eastern practices, nutrition counseling and therapeutic bodywork from leading experts, plus comprehensive analyses of every aspect of a person's health: physical, psychological, spiritual, and cultural. I could not have predicted the feedback I got from clients about their fantastic life changes just a few months into the opening of my new facility. You'll be hearing from some of them throughout this book.

I predict that within the next twenty years we'll see variations of these medical-spa health centers associated with traditional hospital settings. (In 2009 one of my medi-spas opened on the Christus Hospital grounds in Beaumont, Texas, soon followed by another, in Louisiana.) Access to a world-class facility that can treat illnesses using traditional medicine while promoting wellness through programs designed to improve one's appearance and overall well-being has the potential to revolutionize medicine. Imagine a world where we don't affiliate hospitals with illness and disease only, but rather as places to go to reduce cellular aging and, ultimately, restore youth. The Murad Inclusive Health Spa will continue to branch out across the country and the world through innovative partnerships with premier spas and medical facilities. The trained practitioners at these spas and facilities are certified by my University of Inclusive Health to help people customize their own personal programs based on the Water Secret.

As a dermatologist, pharmacist, and researcher, I have devoted my life to making beautiful, healthy skin attainable for everyone. And I have always rooted my practice in the idea that skin care can lead the way to overall health. The skin, after all, is a microcosm of the entire body—it reflects what is going on inside. The treatment I use to heal the skin has a dramatic effect on overall health—so dramatic, in fact, that patients now come to me to be healed in ways that go far beyond the scope of traditional dermatology. They look to me to help ease other unique health concerns by complementing standard care for conditions including arthritis, infertility, fibromyalgia, high blood pressure, insomnia, chronic fatigue, digestive problems, and diabetes with the science of the Water Secret.

How to Use This Book

Of all the works I've written or contributed to, I'm especially proud of this book. Given the leaps and bounds we've taken in the past thirty years in medicine and dermatology, there's so much lying in the treasure trove of human knowledge. It's been thrilling to have participated in the hunting and gathering of that knowledge—from those early days when I went outside the box to create my first acne and antiaging formulas, to eighteen patents later and, more recently, being awarded the International Spa Association's Visionary Award, which recognizes breakthrough contributions to the world of spas and contributions to the wellness fields on a global scale. The accolades that I cherish most, however, come from my own patients and from those who've been changed by my programs and advice. I'm never content until my patients are healed, and because I can see only so many people in my own private practice, I won't be content until every person on the planet has the chance to be healed through my message.

The goal of this book is to show you how to apply the Water Secret to your life in a practical, doable, and economical way. I will cover the keys to abiding by the Water Secret that will (1) prevent and reduce damage to cells so they can retain more water and nutrients and (2) treat and strengthen your cells' membranes and connective tissues. You don't have to incorporate all three Inclusive Health components—topical care, internal care, and emotional self-care—into your life at once. Think of them as three separate doorways through which you can enter a life of optimal health and energy. While part of my mission is to help you successfully honor all aspects of the triad, if you do just one thing differently this week by embracing a single strategy, you will notice a difference. And that slight shift in how you feel will motivate you to do more.

Unlike other books that offer structured programs, this book presents things a little differently. Programs do not last long for most people, and once completed or abandoned, their lessons are largely forgotten. I want to teach you a lifestyle attuned to the optimal way to age healthily. Taking small steps toward change can surely change how you feel, how you look, and how well you really are. I'll introduce the three chief Inclusive Health elements with their strategies early on, and then offer further guidance with a ten-step outline and menu plan that can serve as your road map for putting the Water Secret into practice. If you work the ten steps into your life over the course of ten weeks, you'll be aligning your personal restoration process within the same time period it takes for the vast majority of your cells to "turn over," or renew themselves. What better way to revive your body than to give every cell what it needs to function optimally during the time it takes for virtually every cell to be reborn?

It never ceases to amaze me how my patients have watched their medical problems diminish and, in some cases, completely *vanish*. Among the hundreds of thank-you letters that I receive routinely from those who've taken my Water Secret to heart, there is a singular thought spoken many different ways: "I feel amazing, better than I've ever felt in my life." My patients not only share how their skin problems have cleared up since they started following my program, but how their health—physical *and* mental—is changing *significantly* for the better. Medical problems that had not responded to other treatments by other physicians were lessening. Excess weight was melting away. They reported sleeping better, growing stronger hair and nails, and feeling energy they hadn't felt in years. Just as I had personally observed changes in my own body while following the Water Secret, my patients were now confirming what I had known for years. Their bodies were acting younger, and so will yours.

When you begin to take care of yourself, you are doing a lot more than regaining your health and beauty. You are building confidence and helping regain control of your life when it seems off balance. You'll soon find that it impacts other parts of your life as well. Every person who walks through the doors at the Murad Inclusive Health Spa in Los Angeles soon realizes this once they commence a personalized program.

But since not everyone can visit my center and participate in all it has to offer, I bring you this book. Just as I do for people at the center, I will show you how to take years off your body's age—no matter what your chronological age is. And that will get everyone (including yourself) to notice.

Let's get started.

CHAPTER 1

How Well Are You, *Really*?

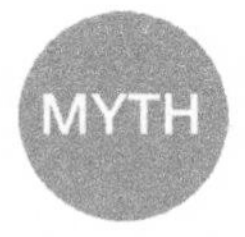

Your weight and vital signs are
ultimate markers of health.

Blood pressure, pulse, cholesterol, and weight are all clues to how well the body is operating, and we're taught to believe that they mean everything. But what if I told you that they are not really markers of overall health?

If you were to ask which marker I'd use to determine how well a patient is, I'd say "Phase Angle" (PA)—a new diagnostic tool used in many research circles to determine the condition of the body, specifically the body's cells. Unlike those other assessments of bodily functions, each of which is specific to a certain part or process, your PA tells you how strong every cell in your body is right this second.

The development of this diagnostic tool played a big part in my discovery of the Water Secret, which is based on how well your cells can stay hydrated to support their life-sustaining functions. The essence of the Water Secret, which I stated plainly in the Introduction, is the following: vibrant health from the inside out lies in *maintaining strong cells that can attract and keep water the way younger cells do*. If you can repair your cell membranes (and I mean *all* cells, from brain cells and heart cells to connective tissue and your outermost skin cells that present you to the world) while attracting water and nutrients to them, you can fight aging and disease. While you won't find PA screenings offered in most clinical settings or at your doctor's office yet, at the end of this chapter you'll find a

Pop Quiz

Which car would you rather drive—a sedan with 200 horsepower or a roadster with 600 horsepower? The roadster, right? But what if it was missing two wheels and hadn't had an oil change in two years?

The Phase Angle test would tell you to pick the sedan.

quiz that can help you gauge your wellness and how you would score on the PA scale that helps measure the integrity (that is, water-holding capacity) of your cells.

The New Science of Age Reversal

When I first conceived of the Water Secret, I was looking for the most comprehensive approach to understanding health and aging. Theories about chronic inflammation and free-radical damage, among countless others, weren't enough for me (the last time I checked, there were more than three hundred theories on aging). In 2009 the Nobel Prize for Physiology or Medicine was awarded to three Americans whose experiments were pivotal in our understanding of telomeres, the protective coverings on the ends of chromosomes that impact cell division. The amount of telomerase, the substance in the body that builds telomeres, ultimately influences cell death and, in the larger scheme of life, aging.

But none of these theories paints the whole picture for me. Certainly these biological events and substances play a proven role, but I sense that they do so within a much larger and universal context.

So with every idea that has emerged on aging, in the back of my mind I continued to hear the famous words of Nobel Laureate in Medicine Albert Szent-Gyorgi von Nagyrapolt:

"Discovery is seeing what everybody has seen and thinking what nobody else has thought." And even though I've led plenty of pioneering studies about the importance of quelling inflammatory pathways and loading up with antioxidants, I have always felt that something was missing. Like a house with a caved-in roof, it does no good to replace it if you don't take care of what damaged it in the first place, such as termites that weakened the structure before the latest storm hit.

> It's difficult to say which theory, or combination of theories, on aging is correct. Regardless of how we age, the net effect is cellular water loss.

Now before your imagination starts seeing termites invading your body and poking holes in your cells (it's not *really* like that), let me briefly take you back to the events that led up to the Water Secret's establishment. My discovery didn't happen in the lab or in a midsummer night's dream. As with many scientific breakthroughs, it evolved over time as I grew to understand my patients and gather evidence from them. It's amazing what you can learn from patients when you delve into their habits and their personal "secrets" to staying young, especially when you witness tens of thousands pass through your office from all walks of life. Some seem to defy their age as if by magic, while others show clear signs of having jumped too far ahead before their time. Genetics and luck aside ("luck" means avoiding diseases of unknown origin and regardless of lifestyle factors), there were clear patterns among those who were aging exceptionally well and those who looked desperate for a reboot.

One patient has always stood out in my mind. When Alfred walked into my office more than a decade ago, he was in supreme health for a man of eighty-eight. He never got sick. He hiked every day, stayed active in community events and organizations, had a positive outlook on life even though he'd lost his wife a few years previously, and enjoyed a healthy diet that included eggs every other day. Alfred may have had good parents, but I knew that his chosen lifestyle more than anything else dictated how well he lived. He was just one of thousands who offered me insights into aging well, and I took his wisdom to heart. After all, I also was looking for the recipe to feeling and looking as vibrant as possible. Patients such as Alfred helped me to see where I could make improvements and then share that knowledge with others.

One fact I consistently observed was that my healthiest patients shared an ability to hold water without the classic "water retention" in the wrong areas. In other words, they were well hydrated (and looked healthy), yet they were not bloated—and they did not lug around bottles of water all day (which, by the way, was not a hip thing to do until recently; some European countries that boast incredibly low mortality rates wonder why Americans seem to have to have drink cups in their cars). My own experience as an avid hiker who continually felt dehydrated on strenuous climbs inspired me to think in this new way and experiment with ways to encourage my cells to hold more water. I theorized that the water-conserving strength of the cell's membrane—its ability to keep water *inside the cell* (hence the term *cellular* water)—was the fundamental marker of health and youthful vitality. The diets of my healthiest patients, including Alfred, were rife with the very nutrients that make up cellular membranes, the outer yet permeable boundary of a cell that envelopes its interior and allows certain molecules to enter or exit the cell.

> Life can be described as a process during which a highly hydrated state of fertilized eggs, embryos, and newborns is transformed into a gradually more and more dehydrated one.

Eager to translate this theory into practice, I used my background as a pharmacist and a physician to attack the problem of cellular water loss. Of course, I naturally became my first case study as I experimented by taking various nutrients in the hopes of creating an ideal environment for maintaining the building blocks of healthy cells. This included supplementing my diet with antioxidant minerals, vitamins, and plant-based compounds; adding anti-inflammatory agents to the mix to prevent free radicals from forming in the first place; and finally, including some omega fats to draw more water to the cells. (And, like Alfred, I started to eat eggs every other day.) My weekly hikes afforded me the perfect testing grounds.

Flash forward several years; by the mid-1990s I was sufficiently convinced that my theory had been validated by my own experience that I was eager to share it with a few hundred patients whose health needed a boost. Not to my surprise, I found that those who took advantage of my internal care program felt better, slept better, and experienced a remarkable reduction in the severity of common skin disorders such as dryness, acne, and cellulite formation. I also found that their skin had an apparent increase in structural strength and resilience that made it appear firmer, plumper, and brighter—more like young skin. And I knew, as every dermatologist does, that outer appearances reflect what is going on inside.

With the help of Phase Angle (PA) technology, which was emerging to measure both cellular integrity and the ratio of water *outside* the body's cells to water *inside* its cells, I further validated my theory. All living things, animal or plant, have a PA. The test that determines a PA involves passing a painless electrical current through your body to ascertain its composition, and from there to make certain calculations. Efficient, healthy cells are the building blocks of a healthy body. The higher your PA, the higher your cells are functioning and the more likely that your cells' membranes are intact (a good thing); lower PAs are associated with cell death or compromised cellular membranes (a bad thing). So when the PA goes up, you're healthy; when it goes down, you're ill. The PA also goes up when you're calm and down when you're stressed. When you exercise more and increase your lean muscle mass, your PA goes up.

PAs have given us a remarkable window into how the body responds to changes in health—for better or worse. This explains why people with illnesses such as HIV or cancer, or

The Phase Angle goes up when you're healthy and down when you're ill. It also goes down as you age. When you increase your Phase Angle, you slow down aging.

those who are nutritionally deficient, routinely exhibit low PAs. As expected, PAs also decrease with age as your body loses its capacity to repair and turn over new cells as quickly as it did in its youth. The true age of a human being can be determined by the changes in the Phase Angle. In as few as four weeks, I've watched patients turn back their physical clocks by following my program. An eighty-five-year-old can have a PA age of someone of fifty; a fifty-five-year-old can have a PA age of someone of thirty-five; and a thirty-year-old can have a Phase Angle age of someone of twenty.

By 2000, I'd hired a research staff and put my theory through more rigorous testing, both in the lab and in a clinical setting. The addition of external and emotional care to my test subjects enhanced their results, and my three-part program based on the Water Secret was born. In the past eight years, we've treated more than two thousand patients and witnessed incredible transformations. Mary, thirty-eight, developed early-stage diabetes as an adult and came to me with a persistent case of acne. A month after following the Water Secret alongside a specific treatment for her acne, Mary's blood sugar stabilized and her acne cleared. Jon, fifty-five, suffered from cysts and depression because he was besieged with the pain of rheumatoid arthritis. Three months after he adopted the strategies aligned with the Water Secret, his arthritis pain was considerably reduced and his depression was lifting. And there was Susan, sixty-six, who, like many postmenopausal women, complained of general aging and skin problems. After ten weeks on the program, her PA placed her at fifty-five years old—more than ten years younger than her chronological age. Each week took back a year of her life, which was clearly visible in a measurable reduction of wrinkles, UV damage, and body fat.

You'll read more success stories in depth throughout this book. There is no reason why you can't become one of them.

In Their Own Words

Before I truly embraced the Water Secret, my life was a mixture of stress, anxiety, depression—and, of course, the good stuff such as family, love, and laughter. My weight was slowly creeping up, my sleeping habits were terrible, and every morning my body ached as if I were an eighty-year-old woman trying to get out of bed. I was a mess. Dr. Murad helped me address my weight (high!) and stress management (nonexistent!), which I'm usually very sensitive about. I've had other doctors talk to me about my weight, but I'd usually get so depressed I would go on a "depression food binge" right after my appointment. But not with Dr. Murad. He gave me hope and confidence. For the first time, I felt that I could get healthy again. It hasn't been easy, but with the tools that were offered to me I'm able to get back on track a lot faster when I veer off. It's been almost two years now and I've kept off twenty pounds and am no longer a screaming mom (well, sometimes☺, but not nearly as much as I used to be). I have more patience with my very active boys, which is definitely a good thing.

—Lori C., forty-one

Where's Your Water?

Contrary to popular belief, you *are not* 75 to 80 percent water. You were once—long ago, when you were a babbling baby fresh from your mother's watery womb. But now you're closer to 50 percent water. What happened? Well, you've aged, and since those early years, internal and external factors have damaged your cells and weakened their ability to retain water. This explains the signs of aging that probably emerged in your late twenties or (if you were lucky) early thirties: your skin began to become drier, fine lines and wrinkles appeared, sleep patterns changed, your flexibility took a hit, digestion slowed, and your energy wavered. You complain about more aches and pains, need more caffeine to get through your day, and have a tougher time keeping excess weight off. This didn't happen overnight, although it may have seemed that way one random day when you "suddenly" noted all these changes in the mirror, on a scale, or in your doctor's office.

What's been going on has been a slow, inevitable decline in your capacity to stay hydrated, which, by the way, has nothing to do with how much water you drink (more on that later). *Hydration* has to do with the water your cells can hold on to for good use. If you drank a gallon of water a day and I called you dehydrated, would you believe me? Probably not. But it's true: unless your cells can retain the water they require to support cellular functions, then all the water you drink in the world won't make much of a difference (and you'll need to keep drinking to keep up with your body's constant cellular water loss). Every part of the body, from your brain to the tendons and ligaments in your feet, needs water to function properly. Without enough water in their cells, organs cannot perform their normal operations or communicate with each other.

This brings me to another fact that goes against the grain of conventional wisdom: not all water is created equal. As you've probably figured out by now, there are two types of water in your body—*wellness* water inside your cells, and *wastewater* floating between your cells, the kind that will age you and make you feel fat and sluggish. Puffy eyes, swollen ankles, and a bloated stomach, for example, are all examples of extracellular waste fluid and signs that the body isn't handling water efficiently. This damage can occur anywhere, including in the blood vessels, heart and other muscles, skin, and liver. Picture a blood vessel that's as strong and sturdy as a brand-new hose. Now picture that same hose riddled with microscopic holes and leaking water. That water escaped and became waste.

Wellness water, on the other hand, sustains cellular activities and thus life; this is what allows you to remain healthy, trim, and beautiful. The caveat, of course, is keeping water where it's supposed to be if those cells are somehow compromised and porous as an outcome of aging. First, you have to sew up those cracks, and then you have to ensure that you're consuming high-quality water, which you won't necessarily find from a bottle or a faucet. You'll shortly come to understand what I mean as I take you through my food pyramid and train you to choose foods and beverages that optimize your hydration.

No matter how much water you drink, it's never enough to keep you hydrated and feeling good unless it can reside *inside* your cells.

Bewitching the Dry Spell to Beauty

When patients ask me to explain how such a focus on water could be so critical, I offer another perspective: you've gone from being a glass nearly full with water when you were born to a glass that's half empty. And a glass that's half empty can't handle the rigors of daily life as well, from those pesky free radicals that swarm in response to certain lifestyle habits and exposure to UV rays and pollution, to chronic inflammation or any other factor that accelerates the aging process. I often find myself fielding questions about inflammation in particular, a concept that has been running rampant in health and beauty circles lately. Millions of dollars and the most brilliant minds in the world have been unraveling the mystery of how inflammation causes your body and skin to self-destruct. But it has caused much confusion among the public, who now seem to think it's a disease itself.

I'm going to dispel many myths in this book, and this will be one of them. Inflammation is a *symptom*—a sign of something else going on in the body that ushers the inflammatory response for help. Think of it as our body warring against harmful agents,

Inflammation is routinely advertised as something bad for you. The truth is that inflammation is a warning sign that the body is trying to heal itself. It's key to survival.

an indication that the body is repairing itself. You would die without an inflammatory response. It's key to the immune system. It tells us our immune system is working. If we never had inflammation, there would be no action within the dynamic cellular immune system network to offer assistance within the body. Knowing this, it becomes clear that inflammation in a healthy body, when it's not an overreaction, chronic, or irreparable, really results in increased general health because of the repair process that's happening at the cellular level.

Here's a prime example to explain: when you cut your finger, the inflammation process begins, ultimately to spur the healing. Once the skin is healed, the inflammation goes away. In the case of more serious forms of inflammation, such as heart disease, which results from a long-term smoldering of chronic internal inflammation, the same holds true. If you were to take care of the underlying cause of the heart disease—high blood pressure or cholesterol, for example, brought on by a poor diet and lack of exercise—then the inflammation would go away, and so would the disease. It's very difficult, if not impossible, to "treat" inflammation. You have to treat the *causes* of inflammation. But treating all of the causes of aging is a mighty tall order. What if you could address what happens as a result of the aging process, and then essentially reverse-engineer the treatment? That's what the Water Secret does. Because the Water Secret offers a unifying theory that helps us make sense of the aging process, it tells us *how to slow it down*—and in some cases *reverse* it—from a singular focal point.

Regardless of what causes aging or disease or even wrinkles, the final common pathway is that there is a reduction in water in our tissues. Yes, we can say that life is simply a slow process of continual dehydration. We wilt and wither over time, just like that plant you forgot to water until it was too late. Even Hippocrates, the father of medicine, thought of the human body in terms of four main atmospheric categories more than twenty-three centuries ago: humid, dry, warm, and cold. He said when we are young, we are humid and warm, and when we age, these two factors no longer prevail—the body moves into the dry and cold categories, which eventually dominate. And as our cells lose their integrity, we become more vulnerable to all those aspects to aging such as oxidative stress (free radicals), inflammation, and disease. It's a vicious cycle: our cells and connective tissues hold less and less water as we age, and we age as a result of that inability to hold onto water. The graphic below helps put this into perspective.

One of the easiest ways to remember the power of the Water Secret is to think of driving a car across the country. You'll encounter some tough terrain along the way, including dirt roads, bumps, and steep inclines. If your tires get little holes in them, they will hold less air and the engine will have to work harder to go the distance. The car will become fuel-inefficient as it chugs along demanding more work from other parts of the car to keep going. Eventually that extra-hard work begins to exhaust your transmission and things begin to slowly fall apart. A good set of tires can make all the difference. And so can a good set of body cells. Everything about you will benefit.

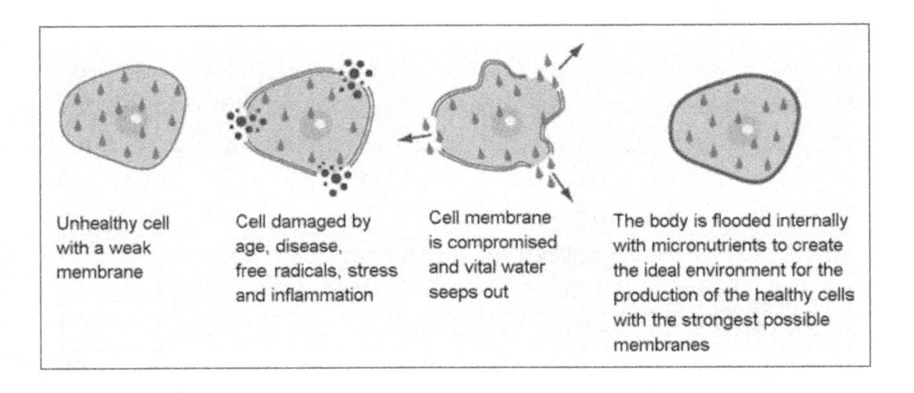

Setting out to find a formula for strengthening the body's infrastructure—predicated on how it breaks down and becomes vulnerable to disease—I discovered the key to the body's ability to act (and look) young. When you take care of your cells' membranes, so they can hold water and support cellular functions, you can effectively fight aging and foster a younger you.

The Water Secret vs. Water Retention

One question I often get soon after explaining the Water Secret is whether people who follow it gain weight due to water retention. True?

Not so fast. In fact, the opposite is true: people who live by the Water Secret *lose* weight as their bodies become more efficient. You will weigh more if the water is in the wrong place—such as puffy eyes or swollen ankles. Water in your cells not only allows you to function at a higher level but also increases your basal metabolic rate so you burn even more calories at rest to lose more unhealthy weight. Here's another way to look at it: as your cells become more hydrated, they function optimally and utilize more energy. In all of my studies of people on following the Water Secret, the one common thread experienced among patients is a heightened metabolism and a reduction in body fat.

Integrative vs. Preventive vs. Inclusive Health

It's amazing to me how many resources we have at our fingertips these days and yet we continue to battle chronic diseases. We have the wonder of powerful new drugs on the market, access to the best that medicine can buy, spalike retreats sprinkled throughout the country, and the knowledge to know the difference between what's good and not so good for us. Yet we aren't all functioning at our best and feeling and looking the best we can be. We're still not 100 percent healthy. Why is this happening?

Integrative and preventive medicine became buzzwords in the past decade. We seem to think that these help solve our health problems, but they in fact perpetuate another problem: focusing on a single condition or disease. Take, for example, heart disease, which is the leading killer in America. If you are a heart patient, chances are you'll be taking medications prescribed by a traditional doctor. You'll be told to watch your diet and avoid unhealthy fats that can clog your arteries. You may even be recommended to an acupuncturist noted for his heart-healthy treatments.

Now, that's all fine and good, but it still puts the focus on a single organ, your heart. What about your stress level and emotional health? What if you've got an undiagnosed problem festering in your lungs or brain that's exacerbating your heart's condition? This is akin to not seeing the forest for the trees.

What I love about the Water Secret is that it not only regards the health of the whole individual but does so by considering every single cell in the body. When every cell functions at its highest level, you optimize your body's environment for the health of every organ and system—not just one. So let's take, for example, the theory about telomeres again for a moment. Like plastic tips on the ends of shoelaces, telomeres sheath the ends of chromosomes to keep them from "fraying" and losing their genetic content. Without telomeres the chromosome and the genes it holds would come apart. Telomeres are necessary for a cell to divide, and are involved in directing the number of divisions. In essence, telomeres have a say in cell life (or death) and how well we age. So how can you protect your telomeres?

Think about it. Telomeres are part of a cell. To protect our telomeres, we have to protect our cells. We have to preserve normal cellular functioning. And that is exactly the goal of the Water Secret. Another way to think about it is to see the Water Secret as the means by which we gain control of our cellular health. It supports optimal functioning of *all* cellular roles, from maintaining telomeres and encouraging cell division to reducing dangerous inflammation and removing waste products and pathogens. It acknowledges and values both the forest *and* the trees, so to speak.

Hence, *inclusive* relates to the whole body and all its fifty trillion cells. Wouldn't you rather address every single cell in your body than just a cluster in your heart, or liver, or brain? Everything in your body is connected. Though it's become customary to see your heart, for example, as operating separately from your brain, both are inextricably linked. So are your toes and eyes, and your kidneys and ears. It's time for a new—inclusive—perspective. If you can begin to view your health in an inclusive manner, then you've already taken a huge leap. Now you just have to follow through and learn how to take care of yourself inclusively. What's more, the fact that the majority of your cells regenerate within ten short weeks speaks volumes to your potential to uncover a whole new you in that same time period. Imagine what new cells operating at a new, higher level can do for you, your looks, and your well-being.

Checkup: Assess Your Wellness

It helps to have a general idea of where your overall health stands today so you can maximize your journey forward and identify where you could be paying closer attention. You can ask your doctor for a Phase Angle test, but since that's not likely to be available to you, I've designed this simple quiz—an adaptation and amalgam of tests I give patients at my health center. While it cannot give you a PA number or tell you exactly the state of your health from a purely scientific standpoint, it can offer a good indication of your general wellness while at the same time revealing alarming insights.

This is unlike other health tests you may have taken because it doesn't ask about your cholesterol level or number on the scale, so don't panic. Be honest with yourself as you answer these questions; don't try to cheat by answering a "right" answer that you think will boost your score. There's no one here but you and these responses. The more truthfully you answer, the more accurate are your results and your capacity to transform yourself starting today. Take your time to think about each question and possible answer. Revisit this quiz whenever you want to see if any of your answers have changed, as a way of checking in with yourself to see how you're doing. Note that you also can log onto the Web site www.thewatersecretbook.com and take an online version of the test that will do the scoring for you and present your personal health profile.

1. I am generally:
    A. happy and healthy
    B. somewhat happy but not as well as I'd like to be
    C. often depressed, frustrated with my health, and emotionally out of control
2. I experience stress:
    A. chronically; it's never-ending
    B. more times than I'd like to admit
    C. only occasionally
3. If my best friend or spouse had to evaluate my stress, he or she would say I:
    A. am moderately able to deal with it, but have my moments
    B. am cool as cucumber
    C. tend to lose it; I can turn into someone else
4. I get more accomplished in the mornings than most people I know:
    A. uh, sometimes; depends
    B. yes, pretty much all the time
    C. never; I'm always catching up and chronically low on energy
5. When I tell people my real age, they are:
    A. amazed; I look younger
    B. not surprised; I look as old as I am
    C. trying not to admit I look older than I really am
6. I spend time with friends:
    A. one or more days a week, no matter what
    B. one day a month—maybe, if I can fit it in
    C. almost never; who has time for that?
7. When I think about the next chapter in my life, I am generally:
    A. excited and looking forward to whatever life brings
    B. terrified; I worry about the future
    C. don't really think about it or care

8. I take supplements:
   - A. daily
   - B. when I remember; occasionally
   - C. never
9. I feel the need to drink water:
   - A. with my meals throughout the day
   - B. regularly; I usually carry a water bottle
   - C. rarely
10. I sleep:
    - A. really well; no problem there
    - B. so-so; I don't wake up feeling refreshed every day
    - C. not so well; I wish I could sleep like a baby. I sometimes take a sleeping pill.
11. I engage in physical activity (e.g., dancing, gardening, yoga, jogging, hiking):
    - A. occasionally, but not very strenuously
    - B. most days of the week; I love to push myself
    - C. rarely; I just don't have the time or the motivation
12. I experience stomach bloating and/or digestion problems (diarrhea, acid reflux, heartburn, constipation, gas, irregularity, irritable bowel, stomach pains, etc.):
    - A. very rarely, if ever
    - B. periodically
    - C. chronically; check out my medicine cabinet
13. I feel my weight:
    - A. is fairly ideal; I'm happy with it
    - B. could use some modification; I've tried to lose ten pounds oh so many times on various diets
    - C. cannot seem to stabilize; I have a low metabolism and hate it. I also hate dieting.
14. When I look in the mirror, I see:
    - A. more signs of aging than others my age; I'm not fully content with my age
    - B. lots of deep wrinkles, saggy skin, and age spots; I hate my age
    - C. a youthful appearance for my age; I'm happy with my age

15. The most important person/people in the world is/are:
    A. my family
    B. me
    C. I can't decide.

Scoring

1. a=3; b=1; c=0
2. a=0; b=1; c=2
3. a=1; b=3; c=0
4. a=1; b=3; c=0
5. a=3; b=1; c=0
6. a=3; b=2; c=0
7. a=3; b=0; c=1
8. a=3; b=1; c=0
9. a=1; b=0; c=3
10. a=3; b=1; c=0
11. a=1; b=3; c=0
12. a=3; b=1; c=0
13. a=3; b=2; c=0
14. a=1; b=0; c=3
15. a=1; b=3; c=0

Add up your points. Then deduct:

- 5 points if you smoke;
- 5 points if you drink, on average, more than two alcoholic beverages a day;
- 5 points if you consume at least one meal a day that's mostly processed.

Which one are you?

40–44:	the role model
25–39:	the average person
11–25:	the struggler
0–10:	barely there

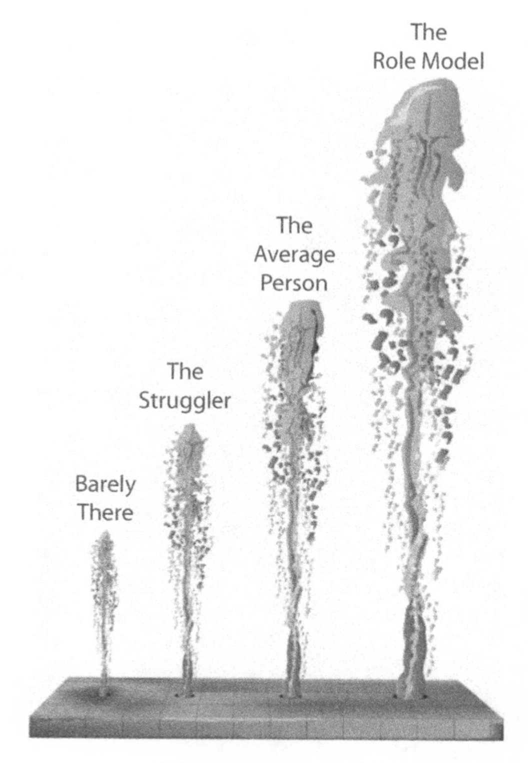

Which one are you?

Clearly, the higher your score, the healthier you are (and probably the higher your Phase Angle); the lower you score, the more you'll benefit from this book's teachings. If you scored below 10, you're a prime candidate for taking every concept in this book seriously and going at whatever pace you need to apply the Water Secret to your life. Bear in mind that it may take time for your body to respond to a shift in your lifestyle, however great or small. Give yourself a breaking-in period for you to establish these habits forever. In fact, some of these habits can create new neuronal pathways in your body. That's right: the brain is not as hardwired as we previously thought. The moment you decide to adapt these ideas to your life is the moment you begin to make physical, neurochemical, and hormonal changes in your body for the better—ones that will support your goal of bringing out your absolute best. Small

Jump-Start the Program

If you want to get going right away with a ten-step action plan, flip to page 89 and follow the steps. You'll need to go review certain sections in the book to gather information, but the plan will give you an outline of things to do to incorporate the Water Secret into your life today.

changes add up and can have a big impact. Virtually everyone can benefit from embracing this principle, including those who would say they lead healthy, happy lives, or who scored above a 30.

Take note of the answers in the quiz that got you zero points. Let those be your focal points as you move forward. For example, you may look pretty good now, but you know that your stressful life is going to catch up with you and start bringing down that appearance and energy level if you don't learn to cope better. I've had patients come into my office and test in the top 1 percent of people who undergo the Phase Angle exam. They are in super shape physically and come close to that "perfect 10." But they know they can always do better, because there is no such thing as a perfect 10. It's simply a benchmark.

No matter where you are on the spectrum of health, remember that you've picked up this book for a reason. A little voice inside your head is telling you that it's time to make a change. Whatever that change may be, understanding the Water Secret will be your launching pad.

CHAPTER 2

Three Kinds of Aging and a Three-Pronged Approach to Care

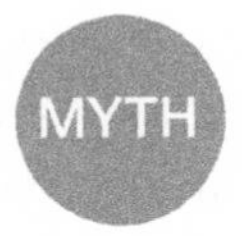

You cannot slow down the aging process.

I'm doomed to be fat, arthritic, blemished, and wrinkly. Look at my parents. It's just a matter of time." Or, "I'm going to die of cancer. I know it. Everyone in my family does."

Most people falsely accept signs of aging such as weight gain, fatigue, and familial patterns of disease as the inevitable. The truth: upwards of 80 percent of longevity is attributed to *lifestyle*—not genes. I see this fact played out every day in my practice, and have for the past thirty years. True, aging is a fact of life. But looking your age is not, and you get to choose how fast you age. Even when it comes to the risk of getting cancer, lifestyle plays a much bigger role. The vast majority of women (70 to 80 percent) who are diagnosed with breast cancer, for example, do not have a family history of the disease. The beauty of the Water Secret is that no matter what combination of aging forces you've got working against you, from lifestyle factors to encoded genes, the Water Secret is a way of repairing every cell in your body and reducing future damage. In short, *the*

> By the time you reach fifty, your lifestyle determines 80 percent of your aging process. The difference between a sixty-year-old who looks fortysomething and a forty-year-old who looks sixtysomething is maintenance. But it's never too late to turn back the clock physically and from a cellular standpoint.

Water Secret helps you to reset your cellular aging processes by giving each and every cell what it needs to live young. When you optimize your body's cellular environment, you give your body what it needs to take care of itself.

As soon as we're born, it begins. With every birthday, new symptoms emerge. A new face line here, a stiffer joint there. And when we aren't careful, this inevitable decline accelerates. The door to illness and disease widens. None of us can escape aging. It's a certainty that Benjamin Franklin neglected to add to his short list alongside death and taxes. The antiaging market has fueled the skin care and spa industries for decades as aging individuals continue to seek new roads to youth. And not just youth in looks, but more importantly, youth in how they feel. No one likes to feel lousy even if all looks relatively good on the outside. If you don't have your health, nothing else—not even a youthful appearance—really matters.

In the 1980s, when I introduced alpha-hydroxy acids to the professional skin care industry, women flocked to their aestheticians to exfoliate away their top wrinkly layers. As years passed, we found better vehicles for our ingredients. At Murad we discovered the power of stable vitamin C used in an anhydrous silicone formula and other topical antioxidants, and we started to see remarkable improvements in skin. But there were limitations on how much skin could improve. Regardless of what we did on the outside to maintain results, and no matter how much sun protection was used, we continued to see the gradual changes from aging creep in. It was clear that skin aging involves more than just external influences, so research would have to go beyond skin's outermost layers. These were still the days when aestheticians, doctors, and lifestyle practitioners followed their own divergent paths without considering the value of sharing knowledge or collaborating.

As I noted in the Introduction, my own search for new approaches to help my patients led me to create an interdisciplinary approach to skincare. I had to look beneath the surface of skin and to examine the relationship of the internal aspects of the body, unfolding the mechanisms of inflammation, disease, and hormones to the health of the skin. My research confirmed what I knew instinctively: that making changes in internal health and emotional composition, in addition to therapeutic skin treatments, produced profound results in not just skin health but also total health. Moreover, my continuing work with the Water Secret showed me, through direct clinical examination, that the key to longevity, youth, and health is at the cellular level.

In my quest to find the next "it" ingredient or method that would take us to new levels of rejuvenation, I was faced with the grim reality that there really is no way to stop aging. (Sorry!) In fact, if you were to ask different scientists what it mean to "age," you'll get different answers. We don't even have a clear definition of what that verb even means: to "age." Facetiously, the only thing that stops aging assuredly is death. All joking aside, aging has perplexed us for millennia, and scientists have explored cellular aging ad nauseam. In the process, researchers have presented more than three hundred theories on the causes of aging. It's difficult to say which theory is correct and which is not, as the answer may stem from a combination of theories—some of which haven't even been brought to light yet. Free radicals and inflammation, for example, tell only part of the story.

All of these theories on aging aside, on closer inspection, a distinct and undeniable pattern emerges. It seems that the largest clue to solving the mystery of aging starts small, at the cellular level, and simply, with life's most natural and valuable element, water as the key. When our cells are not fully hydrated, they cannot function at optimal levels, and this leads to aging. When cells deteriorate, disorders, diseases, and death occur. Studies show that the elderly, especially if diseased, have low levels of water inside their cells. My own studies of people at both ends of the spectrum—those in poor health and those in supreme health—also show distinct differences in their cellular water content. Hence the net effect of aging is cellular water loss—which, as you know by now, is the foundation of the Water Secret.

The Wellness and the Waste in Water

Think of your body as comprised of two ingredients: cells and connective tissue. Both harbor and use water to sustain life, so in a sense you can think of your body as made up of cells, connective tissue, and water. That's it.

Cells make up your muscles and organs, including your skin. Though skin cells are not the same as, say, heart cells, their basic traits are the same. All cells have a protective membrane comprised of fats (lipids) and lecithin, a natural antioxidant and emollient found in all living organisms that's essential to cell membranes. Within this cell membrane is a substance called cytoplasm, and within the cytoplasm is the cell's nucleus. The nucleus is the control center of the cell, and damage to a cell's outer membrane is as lethal to the cell as direct damage to its inner nucleus. Both the cytoplasm and the nucleus are predominantly made up of water. Your heart, brain, bones, and outer skin layer are all made up of cells.

Connective tissue is the fibrous material that binds your muscles and organs in place and that connects one organ to another. This tissue has very few cells and contains what's called the body's matrix, which is semisolid matter made of materials such as hyaluronic acid, a water-loving substance that can attract up to one thousand times its weight in water. Collagen and elastin, two structural proteins you'll learn more about later, keep the connective tissue firm and hold its shape. You get the tools you need to manufacture collagen and elastin from the amino acids in the foods you eat. Blood vessels, nerves, tendons, ligaments, and your internal layers of skin are all connective tissue.

As we age, our cells and connective tissue break down. They lose the ability to attract and hold onto all the water they need to function at their best, as they do in a baby's new body. The water that seeps out wanders aimlessly through the spaces between cells and connective tissue. This, as you'll recall from the previous chapter, is what I call wastewater.

Not only is wastewater useless, it also can cause problems. It can build up in inconvenient ways, leaving you with puffy ankles or eyelids. Your body can be full of this wastewater and still be dehydrated because it can't reach the cells and connective tissues where it's needed most and where it keeps your heart, lungs, brain, liver, and skin healthy and vital. Can anything be done about this wastewater? Absolutely. First, it helps to understand what factors into this water loss, and then to take the steps to reduce that buildup of wastewater by repairing your cell membranes and strengthening the structure of connective tissue.

Not All Aging Is the Same

There's only one word to describe what happens over time—age—but there are different reasons and triggers for this process. Let's look at the three main types of aging. This will help you to completely grasp how to address aging.

What Happens When You Age?

- Wrinkles
- Sun damage
- Less hair in some places, more in others
- Poor memory
- Lack of sleep
- Lack of energy
- Poor digestion
- Reduced circulation
- Chronic disease
- and more

Intrinsic Aging: A Fact of Life

In a word, *tough*! So-called intrinsic aging is simply the natural aging process no matter what you do to try to halt it. It's what would occur had you never been in the sun, swallowed toxins, taken a stressful exam, smoked a cigarette, partied past your bedtime, breathed metropolitan air, and so on. It's what would occur despite sleeping in a pure oxygen tank, avoiding smiling to defy laugh lines, or Botoxing your face stone cold. Genetics play a key role in intrinsic aging. If your parents aged well, odds are you will, too. In the body, intrinsic aging results in loss of collagen and elastin, and reduced water content in the cells.

Environmental Aging: Inevitable but Controllable

Extrinsic aging is also known as "environmental aging," a term I introduced back in 1993. Extrinsic or environmental aging is exactly what it sounds like: aging from the combination of injury to your outsides and compromised cellular functions on your insides. Luckily, this is a type of aging that we can control to some degree. Factors such as excessive sun exposure, pollution, smoking, stress, poor diet, and intake of drugs or alcohol contribute to this type of aging.

The classic signs of environmental aging are usually written all over a person's skin in the form of redness, dryness, thinner skin, sagging, wrinkles, and hyperpigmentation (including age spots). You probably can't see the water loss in the cells, but it's there. The good news is the effects of environmental aging can be minimized through both preventive actions and treatment, which I'll be getting to shortly.

Hormonal Aging: Another Fact of Life

This type of aging has gained tremendous attention in recent years, and has no doubt spurred much conversation, especially in women's circles. Hormonal aging occurs as levels of estrogen decline—and starts happening long before menopause.

Do Men Hit a "Pause"?

Hormonal aging in men, called "andropause," also can occur as levels of testosterone decline. Most men experience a parallel version of hormonal aging, which is less talked about in general, but the effects are similar and widely visible when you consider the hallmark signs: sagging breasts (which is pronounced if they are overweight), excessive hair growth in atypical spots such as ears and eyebrows, and thinning hair on top of the head. Estrogen is not just a female hormone; it's also present in men's bodies, made in small amounts as a by-product of the testosterone conversion process. This estrogen helps support bones, a healthy libido and heart, and brain function. As with women, age can precipitate an imbalance of men's natural hormones. Too much estrogen, for example, can reduce levels of testosterone and trigger a loss of muscle tone and sexual function. It also can cause fatigue and increased body fat.

Aging for women begins far before menopause begins. In fact, by the time a woman reaches her twenties, she will have begun to age and her skin will probably show it. The reasons why this happens vary and include many factors, such as stress and lifestyle.

Although the eventual dryness and inelasticity of skin that come with age are inevitable facts of life, the aging process is a cumulative one that occurs at varying rates from individual to individual. Hormonal aging does not turn on like a light switch; rather, it's like a dimmer that slowly brightens as chronological age progresses, and the speed at which it brightens is different from person to person. Most women are all too familiar with the ravages of low estrogen levels: weakening of the collagen and elastin fibers makes them look old as the skin becomes thinner and more fragile; adding insult to injury, there is an increase in facial hair and breakouts, and reduced water content in the cells. In short, they don't look like glowy youths anymore, and there's nothing more frustrating than the combination of dry skin *and* acne.

So why does this loss of estrogen lead to so many skin-damaging effects? Estrogen is your skin's best friend. It helps prevent aging in three big ways: (1) it prevents a decrease in skin collagen in postmenopausal women; (2) it increases the skin's collagen content, which maintains skin thickness; and (3) it helps skin maintain moisture by promoting the production of certain substances in the skin that boost hydration.

Because everything in the body is connected, shifts in hormones through the years can have profound effects on the body. Hormones are simply chemical messengers that travel in the body's blood vessels to target areas where they have an intended effect. These chemical messages, which are tiny in volume, have many large and important jobs, such as regulating metabolism, mood, growth and development, and tissue function. The body's hormonal system includes the sex glands (testes in men, ovaries in women), the kidneys, pancreas, hypothalamus and the pituitary, pineal, parathyroid, thyroid, and adrenal glands. There are many hormones in the body. In addition to estrogen, the most familiar ones include progesterone, cortisol, adrenaline, and androgens such as testosterone. Every organ has certain hormones, and many hormones have multiple functions that overlap. When all hormones are balanced, the body works as it should, organs function properly, tissues are supple and resilient, and skin is youthful. Conversely, the smallest variation in hormone levels can cause great, catastrophic effects all over the body and on skin.

While the study of menopause-related skin issues began in the mid-1990s, well before then I noted many hormonal skin patterns that exist in women. As I began to isolate certain factors and sift through my data, I was startled to find some direct correlations with hormones and skin conditions. All the while, the term "menopausal skin" became quite popular as some of my contemporaries believed that menopause marked the beginning of skin issues due to hormone decline and imbalance. However, I knew this to be completely false based on my patients' and hands-on experience.

The truth is, as we age, so do our organs and glands. In women, estrogen and progesterone production declines. And as I just stated, hormonal aging does not just happen once a woman reaches menopause. The true beginning of hormonal aging occurs decades before menopause sets in and continues to occur well after menopause.

Unlike environmental aging, for which there are clear and wise lifestyle strategies to prevent and reduce it, hormonal aging is the most troublesome to treat effectively. It requires an inclusive approach and a great understanding of the body's systems and complex interactions. That said, I won't ask you to learn all those systems and symphonic interactions. By following the strategies of the Water Secret, you'll be putting into practice the very methods to heal and control hormonal aging. This is incredibly important because one of the chief side effects of hormonal aging is a decline in cellular immunity. As dried-out, aging cells lose their ability to renew themselves and operate properly, their functionality slows down—similar to a used piece of equipment that doesn't work like new. For this reason, women approaching menopause or beyond it become more susceptible to conditions such as cardiovascular disease, cancer, hypothyroidism, polycystic ovarian syndrome, autoimmune disorders, high blood pressure, obesity, and insulin resistance. They become vulnerable to a bevy of health challenges.

Living Long

According to the U.S. Census, there are more than forty million menopausal women in the United States today, with twenty million more baby boomers entering or already in perimenopause. By 2020, the number of menopausal women in the United States is projected to top fifty million. As of the late twentieth century, the life expectancy of women increased to an average age of eighty-one. This means that most women can expect to live more than a third of their lives after menopause.

Die Late, Not Old

All humans experience a combination of the three types of aging to certain degrees. Despite the fact that hormonal aging is the most troublesome to address effectively, fundamentally it and the other two types of aging can be addressed with one simple element: water.

What I love about the Water Secret is that it offers a unifying theory that helps us make sense of the aging process. It tells us how to slow that process down—and in some cases reverse it—from a singular focal point. If water is addressed at the cellular level, then all skin and body issues can be managed more completely.

Why is this so revolutionary? Because for the past century we've been focused on disease treatment, and studying diseases on a case-by-case basis. Only recently has science turned to slowing the biological processes of aging as a way to prevent and fight a multitude of diseases. Some still think of cancer, atherosclerosis, osteoporosis, osteoarthritis, immune dysfunction, and skin aging as unrelated. But that insular way of thinking is beginning to change.

> Until recently the notion of reversing human aging was a mere fantasy, absent from any scientific support. In the past few years scientists have gained tremendous ground on demystifying the aging process and how to manipulate it—forward or backward.

In 2008 a group of aging experts from the United States and the United Kingdom reported in the prestigious *British Medical Journal* that slowing aging is the best way to combat diseases in the twenty-first century. In other words, the traditional medical approach of attacking individual diseases—cancer, diabetes, heart disease, Alzheimer's disease, Parkinson's, and so on—will soon become less effective if we don't determine how all of these diseases either interact or share common mechanisms with aging. It's true that middle-aged and older people are most often impacted by simultaneous but independent health problems, a condition technically known as multimorbidity. I'll see a fifty-five-year-old man with diabetes, high blood pressure and cholesterol, arthritis, gastric reflux, and a history of depression. The number of medications he's taking is mind-boggling. Or picture an elderly woman suffering from at least ten different ailments and juggling an expensive, confusing cocktail of meds every day. What's more, there are other medications that could be taken, but they cause intolerable side effects, and the more drugs she takes, the greater the risk of dangerous drug interactions. Her predicament is not an unusual one.

Two-thirds of people over age sixty-five, and almost three-quarters of people over eighty, have multiple chronic health conditions, and 68 percent of Medicare spending goes to people who have five or more chronic diseases. As a group, these patients fare poorly by any measure. They linger in hospitals longer, experience more serious preventable health complications, and die younger than patients with less complex medical profiles. Sadly, they are often not treated as whole human beings. Medicine attempts to spot-treat each complicated medical problem to no avail, because medicine cannot yet see the forest for the trees.

The authors in the study reported in the *British Medical Journal* point out that a cure for any of the major fatal diseases in life would have only a marginal impact on life expectancy and the length of healthy life. For example, if we cured cancer or heart disease today, what would that mean for the general population's life expectancy tomorrow? Not much, because something else would take people down. You may be able to save yourself from a heart attack or colon cancer, but you won't escape another age-related ailment, such as kidney disease or a stroke.

> The idea is to die young as late as possible."
>
> *—Ashley Montagu*

I agree with the authors of this latest study that the potential benefits of slowing aging processes have been underrecognized by most of the scientific community. It's time for an attack on aging itself. To that end, I hope that the Water Secret becomes a much-embraced strategy in that arsenal. It offers a new paradigm of health promotion and disease prevention that could result in longer, more satisfying lives. Because it doesn't focus on just a single disease or condition, it stands to have a much greater impact on the health and wellness of people who take its tenets to heart. As I outlined in the previous chapter, an *inclusive* approach optimizes the health of the individual based on that person's most elemental makeup: cells and water. While it's common knowledge that with aging comes disease, few people stop to think about what happens when you reduce aging: you reduce disease. You reduce not just the risk factors for disease, but you can even reduce the likelihood that a certain disease will have a maximal effect on you. In other words, when you equip your body with what it needs to function optimally at the cellular level, you effectively shield yourself from age-related diseases, forcing your body to live younger for as long as it can.

Hormone Replacement Therapy: A Good Thing?

Hormone replacement therapy (HRT) is a hotly contested debate these days, especially with regard to the use of bioidentical hormones. Stopping hormonal aging altogether is like stopping the rotation of Earth. The goal is to prevent menopause from occurring for as long as possible, and this can be done at any time from age twenty upward, not just the "perimenopausal" years—the six to ten years before menopause. Because the general population largely misunderstands the role of hormones in the body, most women won't seek preventive maintenance or hormonal evaluation until a problem (usually external) surfaces. The very nature of questioning hormone levels goes against women's ownership of their femininity. To explore hormone levels at twentysomething seems culturally counterintuitive, as a woman's twenties are socially and physically deemed "the good years." But no matter what we would like to believe, in every case the key is to avoid hormone production declines and imbalances. If you can maintain natural hormone production and balance for as long as possible, you will look and feel years younger than other women your age. You'll age better than your mother or aunts did, and you'll experience less disease and skin aging; in essence, you'll grow old, but you'll do it much more gracefully.

Hormone replacement therapy (HRT), which I only suggest for healthy women with specific problems directly related to menopause, can help prevent many of the physical changes experienced during and after menopause. But HRT should only be used as a last resort; so much can be done during those pre-menopausal years (and even menopausal and post-) to stimulate the body to take care of itself. If the body is as healthy as it can be, then it will function as well as it can and all systems and organs will work in concert with hormones in balance. That is exactly the goal of the Water Secret. Another way to understand the power of the Water Secret in relation to hormones is to consider the following. Picture a cell operating at just 40 percent. It's supposed to be producing hormones that the body desperately needs, but it can't because it's not working at 100 percent. Wouldn't you rather flood that cell with the nutrients and water it needs to repair itself and get back to working at full speed than just to infuse the body with synthetic hormones, which don't do anything to repair or heal the body's natural hormone-producing system? Again, my point is that the Water Secret honors the body's innate needs at the cellular level, needs that go largely unnoticed in today's medicine. Improving your cells so each one can carry out its specific function should be first and foremost on the agenda. There's a time and a place for interventions such as HRT or drug therapy, but even when those are employed, they cannot have a maximal effect unless your cells are operating as best

> Myth: Hormonal aging starts in midlife, or just before menopause. Fact: Hormonal aging begins as early as one's twenties—for both men and women.

they can. By applying the Water Secret, we can make every cell function at its highest potential, giving every organ the best components so that it can operate at an optimal level. So even as the ovaries, for instance, are producing less and less estrogen, they can continue to produce estrogen at their maximum potential. To that end, think of the Water Secret as improving the overall integrity of your body, and any additional treatment or therapy as additional support. But how well that additional support will work, however, depends on the intrinsic strength of your body.

A Three-Pronged Approach to Care: An Inclusive Approach

Keeping your vital waters in your cells is the whole point of the Water Secret, but as I've said, this has very little to do with the water you drink. True hydration can originate from unlikely sources. Think of a time when you splurged on a facial or got a massage. Chances are you looked and felt better afterward. Have you ever noticed that after a great night's sleep, or just a catnap in the afternoon, you looked fresher in the mirror? How about the last time you went on vacation and came back looking younger and feeling more energetic? This brings me to my three-pronged approach to care, the three inclusive areas on which to focus that embody the Water Secret.

For decades, people have been trained to automatically think "diet" and "fitness" when it comes to optimizing health and well-being. The time has come to reposition these two obsolete categories and create a whole new model. Diet and fitness certainly are part of the equation, but I want you to begin thinking of health as coming from paying attention to three aspects of the human self: internal, external (or topical), and emotional.

1: Healing Waters from the Inside Out

It's no surprise that proper nutrition is one of the keys to good health, but what's not commonly understood is that you can maximize your body's capacity to heal itself and support production of robust, healthy, hydrated cells through the foods you put in your mouth. Providing your body with the right raw materials allows it to maintain a healthy water balance, stimulate new cell growth, and repair vital structures. In addition to nutrition, we support our bodies internally through supplements, physical activity (to keep our aerobic capacity, lungs, heart, and entire cardiovascular system strong), and prescription medication when necessary.

Every system in the body is carefully engineered to operate at a certain balanced point for optimal performance. The process through which this balance is maintained is called *homeostasis*. When anything goes awry, the body automatically goes to work to correct it and bring it back to this balance point. This is why you sweat when your body temperature rises. The sweating cools you off, keeping your body temperature at an ideal 98.6° Fahrenheit. If there is damage or injury to tissue your body will innately know that something is out of alignment and attempt to rebuild it from its components. It's adept at rebuilding tissue as long as it has the parts available. Unfortunately, that is not always the case, ultimately resulting in preventable disease and premature aging as damage builds up and goes unrepaired. Connective tissue, for example, is made up of substances called glycosaminoglycans, or GAGs for short. To repair connective tissues, you need to give your body the necessary ingredient—glucosamine. (Much more on this later.)

You also need to provide amino acids, the building blocks for collagen and elastin, which help keep your blood vessels firm and hold their shape. Briefly, the breakdown of collagen and elastin is responsible for the primary differences in appearance between an old face and a young face. But internally, the aging of the blood vessels and heart, sometimes called arterial aging, can be deadly. It's responsible for so many age-related diseases that either reduce one's quality of life or just cut life short: strokes, heart attacks, memory loss, and a loss of blood and nutrients to critical organs. The illustration below shows the progression of damage to a blood vessel. As you can see in the third image, extensive damage changes the structure and function of the blood vessel's walls, rendering the vessel frail and inefficient.

Finally, you need to give your body nutrients to rehydrate its blood vessels and to attract wasted water back to them. The Cellular Water Diet focuses on giving you what you need for every system in your body to function optimally—from the cellular level up. In addition, I'll recommend supplementing your diet with nutrients that are difficult to get in ideal qualities from food alone. This may sound complicated and daunting, but it's actually simple and economical. I'll be going into exact details about which supplements to take in chapter 5.

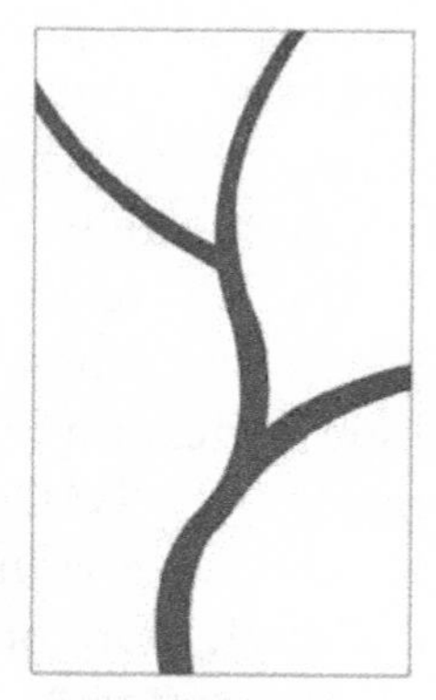
Closer View of Healthy Blood Vessel

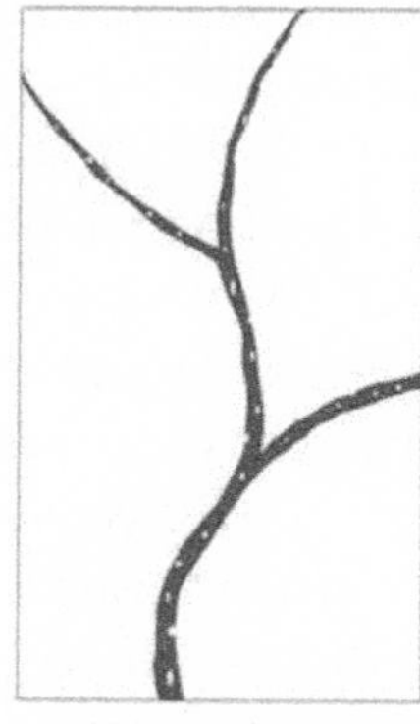
Closer View of Damaged Blood Vessel

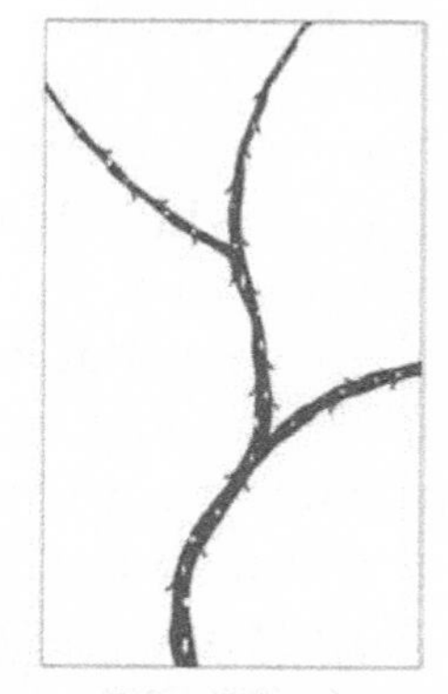
Closer View of Extensive Damage to Blood Vessel

2: Healing Waters from the Outside In

We tend to think of the skin as a separate organ, not related to anything else—a tough wrapping to our more delicate inner parts. The idea that everything in the body is connected is an important concept, though. The skin is connected to every system in the body—from your cardiovascular and digestive systems to your immune, muscular, reproductive, endocrine, lymphatic, nervous, urinary, and skeletal systems. All must work in synergy for total body health. Both heart and skin, for example, rely on veins. This helps explain why, when you get angry, your heart beats faster and your face reddens. This interconnectedness between the skin and the internal body is largely forgotten by people who see skin as a separate entity. It's a two-way street. When we damage the skin, we damage our insides. Similarly, what we experience inside our bodies could have manifestations on the outside. As a dermatologist, I came to understand this whole-body connectivity early on, leading me to seek more and more solutions to external skin problems by turning inward and including systemic factors in skin health.

Accounting for 12 to 16 percent of the body's weight, the skin is your largest organ, and the first line of defense against assault from pathogens, UV radiation, chemicals, and physical impact. Because it's a visible organ, it's usually the first place we find signs of aging. Looking at it provides a window into cellular and connective tissue health throughout your body. The cyclical process of cellular turnover—the complex phenomena of tissue growth, repair, and breakdown—says a lot about how we age. When we think of aging on the outside, we are really talking about how fast our collagen and elastin—which keeps our skin springy, resilient, and vibrant—deteriorate over time. Once damaged, these fibers lose water and become dry and brittle, leading to wrinkles and sagging. Water in fact is lost from every component of the skin, which explains the difference between a twentysomething's dewy complexion and your grandmother's.

The Skin's Signals

Your skin is not just your largest organ, it's also the most interconnected. Poets call the eyes the windows of the soul, and perhaps they should call the skin the mirror of your heart, lungs, liver, and kidneys. Classic examples of this are the yellow tinge the skin takes on when the liver is in trouble; the red face that can indicate heart trouble; and edema that indicates kidney trouble.

Despite what you might think, there are lots of ways to treat the skin that will reverse visible signs of aging, and help prevent further decline. This includes appropriate topical skin care regimens that you can do at home or with the help of an aesthetician at a spa, and cosmetic medical services—all of which I'll be covering in chapter 7.

Fundamentally, we now know that the key to healthy skin is found at the cellular level and that a youthful outer layer relies on optimizing the condition of your outmost cells, which are constantly under siege by the environment. Healthy skin cells that can function properly and replicate predictably will preserve your health, hold healthy water in, and ultimately slow the natural aging process. People often forget that skin cells need the same constant supply of water, oxygen, vitamins, and nutrients as every organ and tissue in the body. Skin also contains connective tissues that thirst for attention, just like the connective tissues found in blood vessels, nerves, joints, tendons, and ligaments.

Also keep in mind that the relationship between your skin and your internal organs and tissues reflects a similar relationship between your cellular membranes and each cell's internal bodies, known as "organelles." Without the protection provided by the skin, such as is the case in an extensive burn, your body dehydrates, and perfectly healthy internal organs fail. Similarly, if your cellular membranes are damaged and cannot protect your cells, the cell dehydrates, the organelles will stop functioning, and the cell dies. As we age, our stratum corneum—that outermost layer of skin cells—becomes more porous, setting us up for challenges that can go far beyond just our skin alone.

3: Taking Care of Your Emotions

Reducing the negative effects of emotions and stress on the body is key to optimal health. Patients may come to me with specific dermatological problems, but I can't help them effectively without addressing their psychological and social balance in tandem with their skin care. Science is just beginning to uncover the relationship between our physical and our psychological health. And of all the "prescriptions" I give patients to help them to look and feel better, the hardest one to take is for them to give themselves permission to reduce their stress through feel-good services offered at spas, engaging in more exercises or practices such as yoga that combat stress, and establishing support groups to nurture their psyche. In chapter 8 I'll be giving you ideas for managing the stress in your life. I also will introduce the concept of Cultural Stress, which, as I pointed out in the Introduction, is the most pervasive, harmful type of stress these days. My strategies are aimed to boost your self-esteem and allow you—and your cells—to function at their highest level.

Making New, Keeping Old at Bay

The Greek philosopher Plato once described necessity as the mother of invention. Through the years, I've witnessed confirmation of this ancient wisdom in the countless scientific discoveries that began with doctors searching for new and more effective ways to meet the needs of their patients. These findings have shaped, and continue to shape, treatment options, and educate professionals in every field of medicine and therapeutic care.

Despite the fact that aging is part of the life cycle, as is the continual decline in function of all of your body's systems, we are not on a path of decay and deterioration from the day we are born. Much to the contrary, the body is a remarkable machine—continually repairing itself, replacing lost cells and damaged proteins, making new mitochondria and new molecules, and fixing DNA. It is with this in mind that I've designed a ten-week protocol to help you maximize your body's natural renewal system. The "new you" at the end of ten weeks won't be just metaphorical; it will be physical all the way down to your cells, their membranes, and their internal components. Every day your body gives birth to new cells and tissue—out of necessity. Every month your skin cells turn over. Your stomach lining renews every five days, your liver every six weeks, and your skeleton every three months. Imagine the work involved behind those scenes, and the compromises that must occur when the body lacks the right raw materials needed for it to function at its optimal level. As the body ages, it requires an increased quantity of these raw materials; the better you are at supplying them, the more successful you will be at slowing down your aging process.

And there's no better way to dive into the specifics of those materials than to start with a nod to Mother Nature.

CHAPTER 3

Eat Your Water, Don't Drink It

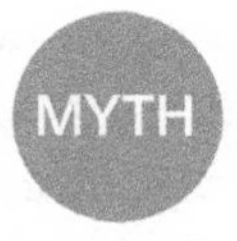

You need eight glasses of water a day.

Most Californians are still asleep at six in the morning when I grab my gear for a trek in the canyons, mountains, and meadows near Los Angeles. The air is crisp. The wilderness is quiet. As the sun rises behind the mountains, dewdrops catch the early morning light on plants at my feet and small sweat beads gather at my brow.

I am reminded of the importance of water and the symbiotic relationship between man and vegetation every time I hike. I've long been interested in plants since my days as a pharmacy student, and the study of ethnobotany in particular—understanding the relationship between plants and people and how cultures use fruits and vegetables that are indigenous to a region for survival. Ethnobotany has been the foundation of my research for many years. Working with pomegranate extract back in the early 1990s, I came to understand the relationship between the fact that it had originated in a part of the world where the sun was intense—and the fact that people had traditionally turned to pomegranate for sun protection. I then set out to prove the topical and internal benefits of the fruit with my own research. Based on my early studies of the pomegranate, we have come to identify other fruits and vegetables that improve sunscreens and antiaging products. Antioxidants such as vitamins C and E have been proven to enhance the SPF of sunscreens; mushrooms are packed with ingredients that can help prevent the breakdown of collagen and elastin, keeping your skin firm and plump; and licorice can help fade discoloration and may help reduce inflammation as well, which can help those with conditions such as psoriasis and dermatitis. The water we consume when we eat fresh fruit and vegetables isn't just any water. It's water that is encapsulated within the structure of food to provide us with a slow and steady infusion as we digest. It's also water that is locked into foods that are rich in antioxidants and other key nutrients, which protect and promote cellular integrity. This is exactly the kind of water we should be "drinking."

In this day and age, we take nature for granted as we walk quickly past bushes outside or bypass fruits and vegetables at the supermarket. For most people, plants fill in the background or are just ingredients in food. What most of us don't realize is that plants all around the world have helped define cultures and tell the story of the human race. For ethnobotanists such as myself, these cultural histories are useful because they suggest new ways of manufacturing today's cosmetics and supplements to improve total body health and skin. They also inform better choices when shopping for the foods that will bathe our cells in nutrients needed for optimal vitality. Imagine transporting a caveman through time and dropping him off smack-dab in the middle of your grocery store. He'd be lost, maybe even terrified, by the strange surroundings and unable to find anything edible among the boxes and packages of products lining the bulk of the store's shelves (unless he tears through a box in his desperate search). If he reached the produce section (often to the far left- or right-hand side of a store), he may feel more at home. Or he may feel bombarded by so many options, and strange-looking fruits and vegetables from the other side of the world, that he might as well be on another planet. And in a lot of ways, he is.

We cannot live without plants. They offer us food, shelter, and medicine. About 350,000 species of plants are estimated to exist. Although researchers have looked at how plants fit in people's lives and how they are used, we are still only beginning to understand the role of botanical ingredients within the human experience. These studies, conducted together by anthropologists and ethnobotanists, have helped reveal a story of endurance where cultures have used their indigenous flora literally to survive. Native healers have shared only a fraction of their ancestral secrets, which are many times handed down through generations and based on ritual and tradition rather than science. Perhaps you can think of some of your own ethnobotanical home remedies passed down from your mother, or learned more recently. Maybe you've taken echinacea for a cold, sipped on chamomile for a good night's sleep, or rubbed arnica gel on a sore muscle. Some of today's best pharmaceuticals owe their origins to plants. Analgesics such as codeine and morphine, and opiates derived from the opium poppy, are just some examples of a class of drugs that gets its power from the plant kingdom. So far, seven plant-derived anticancer drugs have been approved by the Food and Drug Administration (FDA).

Today, science has come full circle and offers clinical data that validate many remedies made by Mother Nature. Because of the global demand for natural and organic goods, cosmetic and supplement manufacturers are increasingly looking at botanical ingredients for solutions. Likewise, dietitians continually push plant-based foods as the foundation for a healthy diet that promises to secure a long, vibrant life. In addition to recognizing the gross nutritional value of plants as a source of minerals, vitamins, fiber, protein, and carbohydrates, science is now focusing on the micronutrients and specialized chemical compounds that make plants especially helpful in regulating aging and disease.

Food Is Medicine

Before there was medicine, there was food. An emerging body of evidence suggests that if we ate a healthier diet, we might not need so much medication. Have you ever asked why certain things grow in some places and not in others? Take, for example, oranges, pomegranates, and apricots, which are grown in the Middle East and also in my own home state of California. These fruits originally came from Southeast Asia, but as people traveled, they carried the fruits with them for quick and easy nourishment. For example, sailors planted orange groves along their trade routes to prevent scurvy caused by a lack of vitamin C in the diet. But beyond ease of transportation and transplantation, each of these fruits served a health purpose. Remember, we're speaking of a time long before lab-formulated vitamin tablets and safe drinking water were readily available, so medicines and hydration came from plants, nuts, fruits, and vegetables, which offered the nutrients needed to live.

Scientifically, we now know that oranges, pomegranates, goji berries, and apricots are packed with vitamin C and other antioxidants, which can help combat cell oxidation and sun damage, and in the case of pomegranates, even boost natural sunscreen levels, which is extremely helpful in warm, sunny climates. Going further, science has illuminated the importance of obtaining antioxidants from the diet because the body cannot make many of them, including vitamin C. Antioxidants also assist in the cellular renewal process and help cells stay plump with water.

What do scientists look for when they study other planets?

Water, because where there's water, there's *life*.

Rewriting the Wisdom

The Water Secret is so simple but so profound: When our cells are not fully hydrated, they deteriorate and cannot function at their peak level. This leads to the tissue damage we refer to as aging. And while this deterioration of the cells ultimately leads to death, before death comes disease, pain, and signs of aging such as wrinkles, inflexibility, fatigue, and loss of mental clarity. Put another way, as we age, we naturally lose water, and it's this water loss that makes it harder for our bodies to heal, free-radical scavenge, defend against invading bacteria and pathogens, and keep the effects of hormonal imbalance in check. But here's the catch: you can't just drink up to replenish your healing waters.

Many people believe that drinking eight, ten, or more glasses of water a day is the answer to hydration. The Water Secret is not just about drinking water, it is about getting water *into* the cells and connective tissue and keeping it there so that every cell can function at its full capacity. If, for example, we want to make cell membranes stronger, encourage connective tissue regeneration (and hydration), mitigate free-radical damage, and keep the immune response intact, we have to flood the body with nutrients.

So contrary to popular thought, hydrating the body is not about drinking eight glasses of water a day, and the best source of water is far from glacial-fed streams. We can drink ten, fifteen, or twenty glasses of premium water each day and never become positively hydrated. If we can't keep the water in our cells, we'll be heading to the bathroom eight, ten, fifteen, or twenty times a day. It passes right through instead of staying in the cells and nurturing the body. That's because the cell membranes are damaged; like a perforated pocket trying to hold coins, the cells themselves cannot properly retain water. The water seeps out of the cells where it belongs and becomes wasted water, the kind that I've already stated shows up as swollen legs and ankles, puffy eyes, and all-over bloating.

> Hydration should be defined by the water you keep, not the water you drink.

I'm not the only one who thinks that the eight glasses of water a day is a sham. In early 2008, researchers from the Indiana University School of Medicine made a list of common medical beliefs espoused by physicians and the general public, myths that either are totally false or lack scientific evidence to support them. They included statements they had heard endorsed by doctors on multiple occasions. The number-one myth listed that has been widely repeated by doctors and in the media was this: people should drink at least eight glasses of water a day.

The study's authors, Dr. Rachel C. Vreeman and Dr. Aaron E. Carroll, found no scientific evidence for this advice. What they did find was several unsubstantiated recommendations in the popular press, which no doubt you've heard as well. The original culprit? It seems that a 1945 article from the National Research Council, which is part of the National Academy of Sciences, noted that a "suitable allowance" of water for adults is 2.5 liters a day. The exact statement was "A suitable allowance of water for adults is 2.5 liters daily in most instances. An ordinary standard for diverse persons is 1 milliliter for each calorie of food. Most of this quantity is contained in prepared foods."

If you ignore the last part of that comment—*Most of this quantity is contained in prepared foods*—you may get the impression that you need to drink 2.5 liters of water a day. Not so. It's easy to get the 2.5 liters per day without drinking copious amounts of water. The most prevalent ingredient in fruits and vegetables is water. Watermelon, for example, is 97 percent water, cucumbers are 97 percent water, tomatoes and zucchini are 95 percent, eggplant is 92 percent, carrots are 88 percent, and peaches are 87 percent water. Foods you'd call dry can also be a great source of water. One slice of whole-wheat bread is about a third water, and a tortilla somewhat more. A roasted chicken breast is 65 percent water, baked salmon 62 percent, and cheeses such as blue and cheddar are about 40 percent water. Beans, grains, and pasta act like sponges when you

Myth: Thirst indicates that you're severely dehydrated. Fact: Thirst should be your cue to drink water, but it doesn't necessarily mean you're technically dehydrated and damaging organs.

cook them, which is why a cup of red kidney beans is 77 percent water and a cup of couscous supplies half a cup of water.

Boiling vegetables leads to water loss, however, because the heat breaks down the cell membranes and allows some of the water to leak out from the plant cells. For this reason vegetables weigh less after boiling in water than they did before, which is why I recommend eating as many raw vegetables as possible.

The Power of Plants

Through good nutrition and healthy lifestyle habits, we are able to build the healthy cells needed to repair the tissues in our body and we're able to improve total well-being. It seems that indigenous people knew this innately. Dehydrated cells are not resilient and do not function properly, and this affects the immune response—but science has only recently uncovered this fundamental Water Secret, as well as why plants can be so powerful.

Picture a ten-year-old girl somewhere in Indonesia, sitting down for dinner. She has lemongrass and coconut soup, a bowl of rice, and a fish stir-fry loaded with locally grown vegetables. She drinks green tea and satisfies her sweet tooth with fruit for dessert. Now whip around the globe to anywhere, U.S.A., where another ten-year-old girl has been called to supper. She joins her siblings at the table for a bucket of fried chicken, mashed potatoes and gravy, biscuits, and pressure-cooked green beans bathed in a sweet sauce made from artificial ingredients. A liter of soda is passed

> Fact: According to the USDA, most people get about 70 percent of their calories from animal products, processed food, and junk food. Only about 30 percent of their calories come from plants. Nearly everyone in nutritional science believes that these percentages should be reversed.

around to fill their glasses. For dessert, she has a slice of cookie dough pie.

If both girls continue on this culinary path, the American has twice the chance of getting cancer in her lifetime, and a higher risk for a slew of diseases, from diabetes to heart disease. Why? It has a lot to do with their choices at the table, and everything to do with what's in those vegetables and fruits.

Phytochemicals Fight On

Researchers call plant chemicals known to provide specific health benefits phytochemicals, or phytonutrients. Some of them will fight both nutritional deficiency–linked diseases such as anemia and scurvy as well as the age-related diseases that dominate our world today, including heart disease, high blood pressure, cancer, arthritis, diabetes, and stroke.

One of my favorite families of phytochemicals are the polyphenols, powerful antioxidants and anti-inflammatories found in raspberries, strawberries, and pomegranates. Pomegranates in particular are loaded with ellagic acid, which is perhaps the most powerful polyphenol of all. Other polyphenol food sources include nuts, whole-grain cereals, brightly colored fruits, vegetables, berries, soybeans, tea (especially green tea), red grapes, red wine, onions, and citrus fruits.

Nuts in particular offer many health benefits, including a reduction in the risk of cardiovascular disease. Walnuts, which have been found in sites of prehistoric human occupation in Europe, are rich in essential fatty acids (EFA), and because cell membranes are made up of lipids, EFAs are tremendous protectors of cellular membranes and cellular hydration. Essential fatty acids are essential because your body cannot manufacture them on its own. You must obtain them from your diet. In topical formulations EFAs help repair the outermost skin layer, preserving cellular water. Studies have shown that of all plants, walnuts have the highest content of total antioxidants. But it's not just walnuts that have tremendous health benefits, it's all nuts. (So if walnuts aren't your favorites, you can skip them and find another nut.) Pistachios, for example, have been shown to reduce cholesterol and triglyceride levels as well as abate inflammation.

Next to polyphenols, another important family of phytochemicals includes the carotenoids and retinoids, the phytonutrient gems that impart so much color to the plant kingdom. Not only are these compounds an excellent dietary source of vitamin A, they are promising weapons in the fight against cancer and heart disease. Apricots contain a high amount and variety of these compounds, which may be the reason practitioners of traditional Chinese medicine have long used apricots to detoxify the body, regenerate fluids, and quench thirst. Studies have also shown that carotenoids and retinoids may play a critical role in gene expression, cellular death, and rejuvenation as well as the immune function. Many experiments show that diets rich in these ingredients have a specific role in defending against cellular aging. The antioxidant beta-carotene is a carotenoid that gives carrots their bright orange color. Once in the body, beta-carotene is converted into vitamin A, a fat-soluble vitamin that has multiple functions, contributing to vision, immune, bone, skin, reproductive, and heart health. Other phytonutrients include lycopene, which gives tomatoes their red color, and lutein and zeaxanthin, which come from green vegetables. Lutein-rich diets are linked to a lower risk of macular degeneration, a leading cause of blindness.

Asia's Influence

Asia offers the West a large amount of data regarding ethnobotany, because in Asia plants, vegetables, and fruits are viewed as health experiences as well as taste experiences. Food descriptions include "invigorating," "soothing," "good for the lungs," and "for better digestion." So it comes as no surprise that some of the more health-enhancing, exotic ingredients such as goji berries, ginger, green tea, and durian may be found readily in Asian markets.

For remote Asian cultures such as those in Tibet and Mongolia, obtaining fresh produce and vegetables packed with vitamin C, polyphenols, and carotenoids was difficult, but the people in these countries found a powerful alternative with native goji berries. Used for more than five thousand years in these high-altitude areas as a longevity and strength-building food, goji berries are attributed to both long life and a good quality of life. The famed Li Qing Uyen, who, according to regional folklore, lived to age 252, consumed goji berries every day! In this same region, locals claim that the most commonly cited side effect of eating too many goji berries is that you may laugh more. Yet, despite the fact that many of these qualities attributed to the goji berry may seem far-fetched, there is scientific backing to the fruit's health benefits. Goji berries are one of the most nutrient-rich foods on the planet. As well as a vegetarian form of protein chock-full of essential amino acids, a goji berry contains five hundred times more vitamin C by weight than an orange. Goji berries contain more than twenty trace minerals, such as iron, copper, calcium, and zinc. The berries are the richest source of carotenoids, including beta-carotene (with more beta-carotene than even carrots), in the world. They also boost the immune system response and healing. Thankfully, you don't have to travel to the Far East to get a handful of these health gems. You can find them in most markets across the country.

Load Up in the Produce Department

By now it should be obvious: there is no better source of high-quality water than at your local farmer's market or grocery store that stocks plenty of fresh produce. The mantra spoken at my Inclusive Health Spa is *Eat your water, don't drink it*. Virtually all food has some water in it, but the most natural whole foods have the highest water content, as well as an abundance of health-promoting ingredients only Mother Nature can provide. Colorful fruits and vegetables, which contain 85 to 98 percent water, concentrate their water with nutrients, thus making it structured—the best form of water for your cells because it stays in your system long enough for your body to put it to good use.

The advice to eat more fruits and vegetables has been around for a long time, but unfortunately it's not well followed. In 2009 a new study out of Queen's University in Ontario, Canada, looked at the fruit and vegetable consumption of nearly two hundred thousand people in developed countries and found that most people don't get their fill. Overall, 77.6 percent of men and 78.4 percent of women consumed less than the suggested five daily servings of produce. The Canadian researchers, who published their findings in the *American Journal of Preventive Medicine*, also noted that low fruit and vegetable consumption is a risk factor for being overweight and obesity, while adequate consumption decreases the risk for developing several chronic diseases.

> Fewer than 10 percent of Americans consume two servings of fruit and servings of vegetables per day.

So why are we having such a hard time eating more fruits and vegetables? It's a question of lifestyle. On the one hand, we are bombarded by processed foods and seduced by their convenience. On the other hand, some of us have been wrongly taught that fruit can cause weight gain due to its sugar content and that starchy vegetables such as squash and potatoes are "bad" because they contain so many carbohydrates. Much to the contrary, fruits and vegetables contain a wealth of nutrients that support cellular health and facilitate the transportation of water into the cells for use. Have you ever seen an obese person who says the bulk of her diet is comprised of natural fruits and vegetables? The complex carbohydrates in vegetables such as squash and potatoes feed your brain and your muscles and even fuel your metabolism (and hence your ability to maintain—or lose—weight). And there's nothing more quick and convenient than fresh produce, which is widely available to most of us with very little effort.

Juicy Foods

We tend to think of food in terms of calories and fat. If you had to rank a list of foods from top to bottom, the unhealthiest being at the bottom, you wouldn't have a problem putting tomatoes near the top and cookies near the bottom. But I want you to try to begin to see foods in terms of how *hydrating* they are, and not whether they are "good" or "bad." Under this perspective, tomatoes still would rank high, and things such as cookies, chips, pastries, and high-fat and high-sugar foods would rank near the bottom. These bottom dwellers are low in water and actually can be dehydrating. When we consume foods that contain high levels of water, our bodies don't have to expend precious water to digest and process those foods. The water we eat goes toward replenishing our cellular water and maintaining optimal cellular functions.

Here's another way to look at it. Sugar, salt, and pure fat—the top ingredients in foods we typically overconsume—have no water in them. And while we do need salt for survival, it can be very dehydrating and toxic to the body when overconsumed. Your cells need twenty-three grams of water to neutralize every gram of excess salt you eat. Processed and fast foods contain large amounts of salt. For the most part, restaurant foods, especially soups and sauces, also are high in sodium.

In 2009, reports emerged about a rise in kids getting kidney stones, which may seem unusual, but not when you consider the huge amounts of processed foods that our kids are eating these days. Eating too much salt, coupled with not eating enough water-rich foods or drinking enough water to help counter that salt, can result in excess calcium in the urine, which sets up conditions for kidney stones to develop. Johns Hopkins Children Center in Baltimore, a referral center for children with stones, used to treat one or two youngsters annually fifteen or so years ago. Now it tracks new cases every week. Virtually all hospitals across the country have noticed an increase, puzzling some doctors but confirming to others the repercussions of a high-salt diet—even in children. Unfortunately, convenience foods marketed to kids and their busy parents are often high on the salt meter and low on the water meter. Some examples: chicken nuggets, finger foods such as little sausages and pickles, hot dogs, ramen noodles, canned spaghetti, packaged deli meats, and candy bars.

Whether the rise in kidney stones among kids can be wholly blamed on a salty diet is still up for debate. A metabolic problem also may be in play, but the message is clear: too much salt has a profound effect on the body at any age, and can exacerbate existing problems.

Fat Flushers

One more thing about fruit and vegetables: they contain an ingredient that can help flush excess calories away from the body naturally, reduce your risk for a medley of diseases, curb your appetite, lower cholesterol, stabilize blood sugars, improve your immunity, streamline digestion, and stabilize your bowel function. It's called fiber, and it's been a hot topic lately because of all the research from prestigious institutes about the role of fiber in a healthy, fit life. When patients complain about slow digestion, I tell them to eat more fiber. Digestion slows with age, and fiber helps keep it up to speed.

Technically, fiber is the part of a food that cannot be digested or broken down into a form of energy for the body. This is why it has no calories and isn't really a nutrient. It's considered a type of carbohydrate, but it cannot be absorbed to produce energy. Animal products do not contain fiber—it's found only in a plant's cell walls, which is why it comes from fruits, vegetables, nuts, grains, and seeds. Put simply, fiber is part of energy-rich, antioxidant-rich, and disease-preventing foods.

The mechanism by which fiber grabs onto calories and sweeps them out of your system is actually quite simple. Fiber works in the intestines to block the absorption of some of the calories from carbohydrates and fats. Think of fiber as an escort that leads calories out of the body. But does this mean that fiber also latches onto things such as good nutrients and vitamins? Fortunately, there's been no evidence that fiber simultaneously prevents your body's ability to retain the nutrients it needs. In fact, the reverse has been shown: fiber can enhance your body's absorption of nutrients.

In 1985, British scientists examined how well iron, zinc, and calcium could get absorbed in a diet containing a whopping four hundred grams of fiber in a mixture of bran, fruit, and nuts. They also looked at the absorption of the same minerals in a low-fiber diet. Not only did their study shoot down the idea that fiber could prevent the absorption of these particular minerals, but it also brought to light the possibility that fiber could increase the uptake of minerals in the diet. The absorption of iron and calcium in the high-fiber group was "significantly higher."

In the past century, we've gone from getting plenty of fiber in our diets to having very little. In the early 1900s, the processing and packaging of food became an enormous growth industry, "freeing" us from the need to grow our food, to eat food seasonally, and to replenish things that could not be stored. We quickly went from eating fresh, nutrient-dense and fiber-rich foods to eating designer foods devoid of natural ingredients and loaded with sugar, fat, and salt. At the same time, our rates of obesity and diseases such as heart disease, diabetes, and cancer exploded. Food processing is now the largest industry in the world. It's a multibillion-dollar industry that removes a lot of fiber and other key nutrients from our diet. Meanwhile, it has managed to inject a lot of ingredients into our diet that can actually hijack our ability to control how much we eat and compel us to eat more and more of the foods that bankrupt our cells. And it doesn't help that the industry's marketing ploys are quite enticing and convincing.

Fortunately, you can make good decisions in rediscovering nutrition and fiber in your food, and you don't have to give up delicious taste to do so. Most people would do well to get at least 30 to 35 grams of fiber a day. This can be hard to accomplish if processed food is the norm, or if animal products outpace fruits, vegetables, and whole grains in the diet. With the Cellular Water Secret Diet, it's quite easy.

Secrets to Getting More Fiber

One of the easiest ways to eat more fiber is to start the day with a high-fiber breakfast. A bowl of steel-cut or old-fashioned oatmeal with a tablespoon or two of flaxseed meal can pack a powerful punch of fiber. Add to that some blueberries, half a banana, and a few crushed walnuts and you'll be set for hours. Some additional tips:

- **Read labels:** A food label can say it's "a good source" of fiber if it contributes 10 percent of your daily value of fiber, which is only about 2.5 grams, because the current daily value is low (25 grams). A label can claims the food is "rich in," "high in," or an "excellent source of" fiber if it provides 5 grams of fiber per serving. Some whole-grain cereals (for example, Nature's Path and Kashi cereal brands) have high-fiber varieties.
- **Eat the skins of fruits and vegetables:** The skins of apples, peaches, potatoes, and zucchini, for example, contain the lion's share of the fiber, so don't peel them off.

Seventy-Five Ways to Eat Your Water

My favorite fruits (raw and fresh, unsweetened, frozen). Go organic wherever possible, but be sure to always buy organic with those marked with an asterisk because those can contain high levels of pesticides when grown conventionally:

- Apples*
- Apricots
- Avocados
- Bananas
- Blackberries
- Black currants
- Blueberries
- Cantaloupe
- Cherries*
- Cranberries
- Elderberries
- Figs
- Goji berries
- Grapefruit
- Grapes (purple, red, green; go organic if imported*)
- Hawthorn berries
- Honeydew melons
- Kiwis
- Mangoes
- Mulberries
- Nectarines*
- Oranges
- Papayas
- Peaches*
- Pears*
- Pineapples
- Plums
- Pomegranates
- Prunes
- Raisins
- Raspberries
- Strawberries*
- Tangerines
- Watermelon

My favorite vegetables (raw and fresh, unsweetened, frozen, lightly cooked). Again, go organic whenever possible, but be sure to choose organic varieties of those marked with an asterisk:

- Artichokes
- Arugula
- Asparagus
- Beets
- Bok choy
- Broccoli
- Broccoli sprouts
- Brussels sprouts
- Cabbage (green and red)
- Carrots
- Cauliflower
- Celery*
- Collard greens
- Corn
- Cucumbers
- Garlic
- Ginger
- Green beans
- Jicama
- Kale
- Lettuce*
- Mustard greens
- Onions (white, red, and green)
- Parsley

Parsnips
Peas
Peppers* (green, yellow, orange, red)
Potatoes* (white, yellow, red, purple)
Pumpkin
Radishes
Seaweed
Shallots
Spinach*
Squash (winter, butternut)
Sweet potatoes/yams
Taro
Tomatoes
Turnip greens
Watercress
Wax beans
Zucchini

Six Ways to Slash Salt, Boost Flavor, and Hike Hydration

If there's one thing I can't do without, it's herbs and spices to season food. But as you know by now, I'm not a fan of the all-time classic seasoning—salt! Although every cell in your body needs salt (sodium) to work properly, it is ubiquitous in the modern diet, so the chances of being deficient are nil, and most of us consume far more than we need. Salt is essential for the healthy function of nerves and muscles, including your heart, but your body requires a precious concentration of sodium. That's why when we take in extra salt, we require extra water to reduce the sodium concentration to an optimal level (i.e., it's that homeostasis in action again), which results in excess water retention throughout the body. Instead of using salt, try seasoning your meals with herbs such as basil, oregano, and rosemary. These have anti-inflammatory properties, so they act like little anti-agers in your body.

Stock up on the following six spices and see how many recipes you can sneak them into for more flavor:

Ginger: This pungent healer's benefits date back thousands of years. People have sworn by ginger's healing powers for millennia; the Greek philosopher Pythagoras promoted its digestive value, and King Henry VIII of England believed

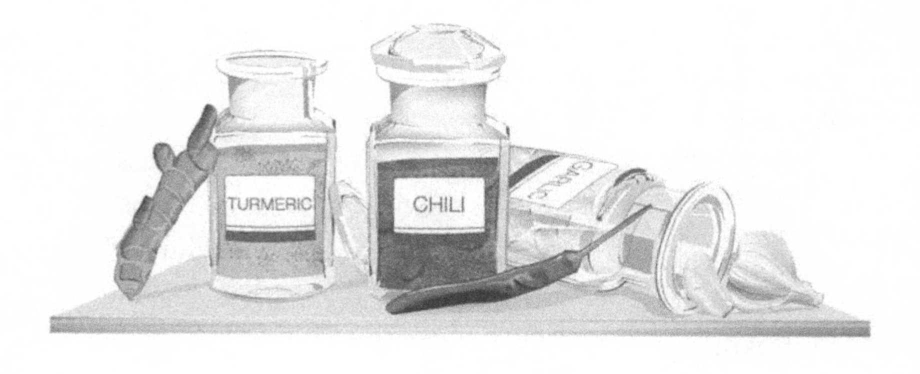

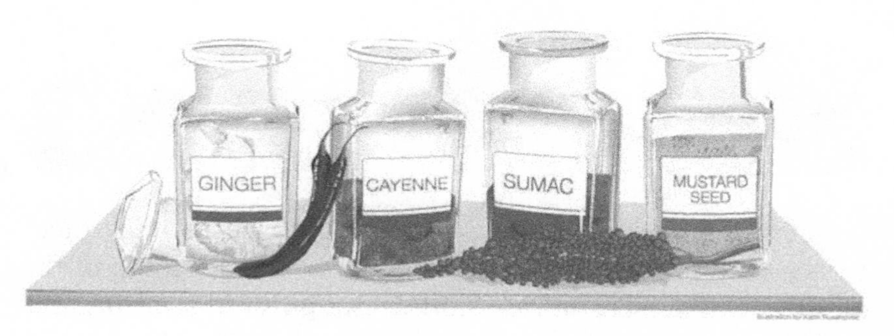

Spices for Life: Traditional Healing Herbs and Spices

it protected against the plague. While we know it won't do much to cure the plague, ginger has been shown to help relieve myriad conditions, from motion sickness to migraines, from high blood pressure to high cholesterol, from arthritis to lethal blood clots. *Tip*: Buy fresh ginger (as opposed to dried and powered) from Africa or India, which will be more potent than ginger from Jamaica. Grate ginger into marinades for meat, chicken, and fish.

Turmeric: This ancient Indian spice found in curry dishes is famous for its yellow coloring, which comes from an agent called curcumin. Studies suggest that curcumin may prevent cancer by virtue of its antioxidant properties and can inhibit cancer cells from growing blood vessels. In animal studies it's been shown to reduce the risk of colon cancer by 58 percent. Curcumin also is being studied for its preventive qualities in treating Alzheimer's disease, arthritis, and diabetes. *Tip*: Add turmeric to curry and Middle Eastern dishes.

Curcumin, the therapeutic ingredient in turmeric, is a potent anti-inflammatory and anti-oxidant; research suggests that, like nonsteroidal anti-inflammatory drugs, it inhibits the action of chemicals that increase inflammation. Animal studies have discovered that curcumin quells inflammation in exercise-damaged muscles.

Chili peppers: Chili peppers and their powder forms owe their mouth-tingling heat source and health benefits to a compound called capsaicin, which is produced by the pepper membranes and then drawn into the seeds. These hot healers have a long history as natural remedies for colds and related symptoms such as coughs, congestion, bronchitis, and sinus infections. From a chemical standpoint, capsaicin is similar to a drug called guaifenesin, which you'll find in many over-the-counter and prescription cold remedies. Dieters have used chili to cut calories and food cravings, including curbing the desire for sweet foods (after all, a doughnut isn't so appealing after you've eaten a hot chili pepper!). Now there's evidence to show that hot peppers can prevent stomach ulcers and reduce the risk of high blood pressure, stroke, and heart disease. *Tip*: Don't be afraid to buy fresh hot chilies and use them in cooking. Examples (from low to high on the heat meter): Anaheim, poblano, green, jalapeño, serrano, cayenne, habañero. Just be sure to store them in paper bags or wrap them in paper towels rather than plastic. Plastic bags can cause them to spoil quickly. Handle with care! The oils from these peppers will stick to your skin, so when cooking with anything hotter than a jalapeño, use caution and disposable gloves (and I'd avoid mixing your own powder in your daily coffee grinder or blender, no matter what your recipe says to do). Sprinkle chili powder in Mexican-inspired dishes, sauces and salsas, chili dishes, and marinades for grilling meat, chicken, and fish. You also can find hot pepper or chili sauces to drop into soups, sauces, and marinades.

Garlic: The benefits of garlic are well documented, and its rewards also date back thousands of years. Multiple studies have shown that it lowers cholesterol and triglycerides and thins the blood, which can help prevent high blood pressure, heart disease, and stroke. People who consume lots of garlic have fewer cancers of the stomach and colon than those who don't eat much garlic. Garlic also is a proven antibacterial and immune-booster, and can reduce high blood sugar levels. *Tip*: Expand garlic's surface area by mincing, crushing, dicing, or eating it raw. This will release the maximum number of healthful compounds. Don't overcook garlic or you can destroy some of its delicate compounds; add it in last to a stir-fry medley of vegetables and olive oil, for example. Watch out: it can burn quickly, and burned garlic isn't very tasty.

Sumac: This spice may not be familiar to many people, and hopefully you don't mistake it for poison oak. The two are related, but the spice is harmless. Much to the contrary, sumac the spice is derived from the berry of a plant called *Rhus coriaria,* which grows in the Middle East and parts of Italy. Sumac is often referred to as the "souring agent" thanks to its lemony-tart and astringent taste. It's long been used to calm the stomach, and today it's seen as a condiment in Middle Eastern restaurants, much like salt and pepper. *Tip*: Try a sprinkle of sumac on grilled meats, chicken, and fish, as a dash over salad dressings, or as a seasoning for rice. It complements lentils and other beans as well as vegetables. In any dish on which you might squeeze fresh lemon juice, go for sumac instead. If you enjoy hummus, top it with an elegant sprinkling of sumac. It's delicious.

Mustard seed: The "mustard" you squeeze from a bottle or scoop out of a jar is actually a combination of mustard seeds and other ingredients, chiefly vinegar, water, and some sugar and salt. Mustard seeds come from the mustard plant, which is a cruciferous vegetable related to broccoli, Brussels sprouts, and cabbage. While there are approximately forty different varieties of mustard plants, there are three principal types used to make mustard seeds: black, white, and brown mustard. Black mustard seeds have the most pungent taste, while white mustard seeds, which are actually yellow in color, are the most mild and are the ones used to make American yellow mustard. Brown mustard, which is actually dark yellow in color, has a pungent, acrid taste and is the type used to make Dijon mustard. Mustard was used in ancient Greece and Rome as a medicine and a flavoring. By A.D. 800 the French were using mustard as an enhancement for drab meals and salted meats. It was one of the spices taken on Spanish explorations during the 1400s. Mustard seeds are a very good source of selenium and omega-3 fatty acids. They also are a good source of phosphorus, magnesium, manganese, dietary fiber, iron, calcium, protein, niacin, and zinc. Mustard seeds' hot and spicy flavor enhances red meat, fish, fowl, sauces, and salad dressings. Whole mustard seeds are often used in pickling or in boiling vegetables such as cabbage or sauerkraut. Brown mustard seeds are an important flavoring in Indian dishes. *Tip*: Keep whole and ground mustard seeds in your spice rack. In India, the whole seeds are often toasted until they split open much like popcorn does. Beware of overcooking the seeds, as they will burn and turn bitter. Since heat causes the pungent flavor of mustard to dissipate, mustard is generally added near the end of the dish and gently heated.

Don't buy spices in bulk. The fresher the spice, the more flavorful they taste. Keep small quantities of them, and replenish them as you use them.

Cleaning out your kitchen and pantry and restocking it with fresh ingredients can be an exhilarating and motivating experience. You may even feel inspired to toss out foods that have been contributing to an unhealthy eating pattern, such as lard, margarine, dry and dehydrating snack foods, low-fiber/high-sugar cereals, refined bread, corn syrup–driven sauces and condiments, and packaged goods that seem to have an oddly long shelf life. If you get into spring-cleaning mode and want to keep going, I suggest also taking a good look at potentially toxic items lurking among your household products.

Clearing the Air

The Green Movement is well under way, but living with pollution is certain to affect most of us in our lifetime. In June 2006 the World Health Organization (WHO) reported that nearly a quarter of global disease is caused by environmental exposures. In what may be the most comprehensive study yet performed to examine how environmental factors contribute to disease and ill health, the WHO stated that of the 102 major diseases reported yearly, a whopping 85 are partly caused by environmental factors. The WHO also stated that we can prevent much of this environmental risk by taking certain precautions and reducing our exposure to known toxins, some of which are an inevitable reality of our era.

If I could transport myself back just a few hundred years, I bet I wouldn't see so much environmental damage to people's skin, and there wouldn't be such a strong need to address environmental aging as today. Toxins, whether consumed or absorbed through the air in our lungs, skin, and eyes, act like little cannonballs on the body, beating it down and compromising systems when those toxins reach acute levels. Toxins also can accelerate free-radical damage and stress organ function—all of which weakens cells and connective tissue, dragging cellular water levels down.

The air is more toxic indoors than out, even for metropolitan residents with high-rises, highways, and industry in plain view. We are just beginning to understand the effects of pollution on our health and vitality, and I'm not talking about the usual suspects of pollution such as belching smokestacks, car exhaust, smog, vapors from gas pumps, oil spills in the ocean, and trash thrown into water reservoirs. I'm talking about the rise in invisible and silent pollutants that we live with every day as a result of modern amenities and technology. These include potentially harmful airborne by-products from electronics, toys, furniture, carpets, upholstery, stains and varnishes, cleaning agents, paints, heating and air-conditioning units, and treated woods. Plastics in particular have taken a major hit lately, as reports have surfaced about toxic by-products that leach from the plastic and into our drinks and foods. One chemical in particular, bisphenol A (BPA), is used to make a wide variety of plastic goods and to line metal foods and drink cans. It's also associated with birth defects of the male and female reproductive systems.

Clearly, the subject of toxins and pollutions can cover an entire book. It's a vast area of study; the Centers for Disease Control and Prevention feels so strongly about the connection between environmental factors and disease that it has created an entire department dedicated to investigating environmental exposure and disease. People also are gaining awareness, and the topic of toxins has come to the forefront of the general public's attention alongside the issue of global warming.

The strategies in this book will inherently reduce your exposure to toxins and help shield you from environmental aging. You don't have to go on a harsh detox diet or cleanse to achieve dramatic results. In fact, I discourage my patients from embarking on any such detox program or "master cleanse." Your kidneys and liver are charged with that duty (to

Body Detox

Your body is the best detox product you have, and there's no such thing as a magical food to purge your body of toxins. But certain foods can help optimize your body's natural purification system. These include cruciferous vegetables such as broccoli, cauliflower, and kale, all of which contain compounds that help the liver break down harmful forms of estrogen for safe elimination. Onions, leeks, chives, garlic, and shallots are rich in sulfur to fortify detox pathways in the liver. Plants from the thistle family—artichokes, dandelions, and burdock—enhance liver function by upping bile flow.

filter out and neutralize any substance that creates irritating and/or harmful effects in the body), and so is Mother Nature's cornucopia of disease-preventing and -fighting ingredients. They've always been there—you just have to invite them into your life and let them do their job.

That said, let me share with you a few additional strategies beyond general nutrition to reduce your exposure to environmental pollutants. I know that the thought of reconfiguring your entire way of living can feel overwhelming, but it doesn't have to be. I'm not going to ask you to throw away your cell phone because it may raise your risk for brain cancer, and I understand that there are pragmatic, economical factors to consider. This is why I love this simple list of things to think about and do as best you can.

Breathe fresh air and drink clean water: It's easier than you think to clean up the air you breathe and the water you drink. Open windows and get some cross-ventilation going for at least thirty minutes a day. Consider investing in an air purifier for your home, or just a portable one for heavily used rooms. Use plants that help filter toxins from your household air and add oxygen. Examples include spider plants, the areca palm, bamboo palm, rubber plant, chrysanthemums, aloe vera, ferns, ivy, and philodendrons. Buy a water filter for your kitchen faucet or just a pitcher that filters water and that you can refill. When you want to take water with you, store it in a stainless steel container rather than a plastic bottle.

Begin to buy natural products: The next time you need to buy a new set of sheets, bottle of household cleaner, or even furniture, try to purchase goods made with natural materials and ingredients.

Opt for organic or all-natural whenever possible: Organic foods routinely test higher on the nutrient meter as compared to their conventionally grown counterparts. As these foods become more widely available to meet demand, they are also becoming more affordable. Remember to always buy organic varieties of the fruits and vegetables noted with an asterisk on pages 74–75, and try to purchase organic meats and fish whenever it meets your budget. Fish in particular can harbor high levels of mercury and other contaminants when they are farmed rather than caught fresh. (For a reference guide to buying fish, see the Monterey Bay Aquarium's Seafood Watch Web site at www.montereybayaquarium.org; some fish are safe to eat every day, while others are more of a concern.) Going organic also will help you to automatically limit your consumption of processed and refined foods, most of which are filled with excess sodium, sugar, and unhealthy fats. You also will reap the same benefits of the natural chemicals that plants have originally made for their own protection. Remember, plants use phytochemicals to protect themselves from disease and to boost their own immunity. They pass those phytochemicals on to you when you consume them. Because organic foods are raised without pesticides, they are forced to produce more of their own protective substances.

Cook and store in nontoxic housewares: Avoid nonstick pots and pans when you cook. Use nonplastic containers and wrappings such as ceramics, porcelain, glass, and natural parchment paper. When heating something in the microwave, ditch the plastics and use a microwave-safe dish covered with a paper towel.

Boost beneficial bacteria and enhance digestion: About a hundred trillion bacteria live in our intestinal tracts (yes, they outnumber our cells!), and some of these bacteria are highly beneficial. They help with digesting some vitamins and they play a big role in our immune response. You are probably familiar with probiotics, the "good" bacteria in yogurt and other fermented foods that can help keep your intestinal bacteria (sometimes called "gut flora") balanced. If you're not a fan of yogurt or other foods with active cultures, you may want to try taking a probiotic supplement to help your body destroy bad bacteria and keep a fine balance in your system that will further help you absorb the nutrients you need so your natural detoxification process continues to run smoothly.

Researchers are currently looking into how *pre*biotics also play an important part in our health. Prebiotics are a class of nondigestible food ingredients that essentially act as food for bacteria in the gut. As they move through the digestive tract, prebiotics are fermented in the colon by the bacteria that live there; this fermentation produces fatty acids that deliver fuel and energy to the cells of the gut and to the good bacteria. This process also inhibits the growth of bad bacteria such as E. coli.

What makes a good prebiotic? Not surprisingly, certain types of fiber, notably those in bananas, berries, barley, chicory root, garlic, legumes, oats, onions, and wheat. The antioxidant chemicals in plant-based foods also seem to foot the bill. These include unpeeled produce (remember that the peel is often the most fibrous part), dark chocolate, herbs and spices, legumes, red wine, and tea.

In Their Own Words

I have been heavy all of my life and my eating habits, though they have improved over the years, were never exceptional. When my daughter was six months old, I weighed 206 pounds at 5 feet tall. I didn't want my daughter's memories of me being about my weight. I wanted her to see me as energetic and active. I wore a size 20 and had to shop primarily at plus-size stores. My feet hurt, my lower back hurt, I was suffering from headaches constantly, and I was not sleeping well at night. I was unhappy with my body and health, and would get stressed very easily. I had a hard time getting down on the ground to play with my daughter. I wanted to set a better example for her and get her started with good eating habits as soon as she was eating solid food. But most of all, I just wanted to feel better.

Dr. Murad's medical center helped me to make the changes I needed. My Phase Angle was low, clearly reflecting exactly how terrible I was feeling. His team gave me a specific eating and exercise plan, the former of which was all about "eating my water," and the latter of which entailed strength training and Pilates classes. I scheduled a massage or a facial once a month (and an occasional pedicure).

More quickly than I could have imagined (seven months), I lost 40 pounds! I started to crave healthier foods. Before I changed my eating, food tasted very blah. Nothing excited me. After a few weeks of changing what I was eating, food started to taste wonderful again. Just plain vegetables tasted great (imagine that!). My feet and back stopped hurting, and I don't suffer from constant headaches anymore. I sleep better and I have so much more energy. Now I can't wait to get home every night and chase my daughter around as she crawls on the floor.

One thing that really surprised me was how much more at ease I became. I don't stress or worry as much as I used to (about anything). I feel like I can take whatever comes my way. Because of my success in this, I'm inspired to set goals in other parts of my life and feel more confident that I can reach them (and have). Not only have I benefited, but so has my family. I have wonderful tools to share with them as well as my friends

(*continued*)

who are looking to improve their overall lives. My husband was so inspired by my success and overall improvement that he also started following my lead and has lost 30 pounds. He gets massages on a regular basis and is much more relaxed in general.

—Amie K., forty-five

Small Shifts, Big Results

Changing the way you eat and buy goods may take some time to get used to. I won't sugarcoat the reality: if you've been eating processed, packaged foods regularly for years, shifting how you eat won't happen overnight. And that's okay. Make it a goal to just change one thing this week in your household. If the thought of depriving yourself of the foods you currently enjoy doesn't sit well with you, then simply pick up more fruits and vegetables at the market and don't change anything else. Make *additions* rather than deletions to your lifestyle at the start. You can and will wean yourself from sugary, fatty foods once you begin to incorporate nutrient-dense alternatives into your life. Your taste buds will begin to change and you'll find yourself obsessing less over the displays at the bakery and more over the colorful array of goods in the produce section of a market. You'll start to order food differently in restaurants and be more conscious about reading labels and asking questions about how your meals are prepared.

Chapter 5 will help you to see the bigger picture of where your diet should be headed. I'd prefer not to use the word "diet" because more than anything, following the Cellular Water Secret Diet is not just a way of eating. It's a lifestyle.

But before getting to my specific nutritional recommendations, in the next chapter you'll find a ten-step guide to putting the Water Secret into practice and daily meal plans to make it easy to start shifting your diet toward cellular health foods. On the other side of chapter 4 you'll find more information to make the program come alive for you.

CHAPTER 4

Ten Simple Steps to Living by the Water Secret: Meal Plans and Recipes

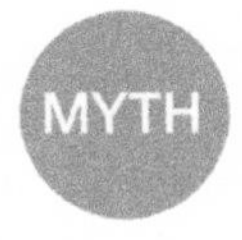

Cells don't renew themselves quickly or easily.

At this point in the book you're probably wondering how to take all the information I've given you thus far and incorporate the ideas into your life right away. It's easy. Just take it one day, one week at a time and use the following ten simple steps to begin making slight shifts in your lifestyle. In subsequent chapters I'll be going into more details about what you're doing, and help you further customize my recommendations for your life and lifestyle.

You can begin to apply these steps however you wish. Do just one a week over the course of ten weeks, adding a new one at the start of each week, or see if you can implement a couple of these today and proceed as is most comfortable for you. Ideally, try to execute all ten steps within the course of ten weeks to see and feel the full impact of the Water Secret. Ten weeks is a key period because virtually every cell in your body is renewed within a ten-week period (often called cellular "turnover"). When you follow the Water Secret program to optimize your body's environment, you're protecting and promoting cellular heath so that your body can build the strongest possible population of cells. At the end of ten weeks you will have truly repaired, refreshed, and rejuvenated nearly your entire cellular makeup from the inside out. Remember, my goal is not to put you on a traditional "program" that has you committing to an unrealistic regimen for a specific period of time and then abandoning it. I simply want you to make slight shifts in what you've already been doing. This is supposed to be easy, practical, and most of all, fun. You'll find that a lot of these steps have the effect of reducing your stress and taking the edge off your brain's daily load of processing negative thoughts. Eighty percent of health resides in the brain, so anything that helps relieve unnecessary stress and creates an environment of maximum well-being will go a long way toward keeping you hydrated, young, energetic, and disease-free.

Step 1: Eat Your Water to Fill Up the Cellular Tanks

If you commit to do just one thing differently this week, start by adding more fresh fruits and vegetables to your diet. Pick three from the list on pages 74–75 that you've never had or haven't had in a long time, and put them on your grocery store list. Include them in your meals and snacks. You can take it up a notch by avoiding processed foods, including fast and fried foods, and artificial ingredients. Don't eat out this week. Eat clean! The meal ideas and recipes in this chapter will help you to achieve that.

Remember: Water loss is the final common pathway to all aging, disease, and wrinkles.

Step 2: Hydrate with Supplements That Contain Key Cell-Fortifying Ingredients

In chapter 5 I'll cover the often confusing subject of supplements. In the meantime, be sure to pick up the following key supplements and take them during or after you've eaten your breakfast.

The Core Four

- Multivitamin
- Fatty acid supplement that contains at least 500 mg omega-3
- Lecithin supplement with 2,000 mg
- Glucosamine (1,200 mg of either glucosamine sulfate or glucosamine hydrochloride)

The (Highly Recommended) Bonus Add-ons

- High-potency B complex: Look for a formula that contains all eight essential B vitamins (see page 153).
- Calcium with vitamin D: Look for a supplement that contains at least 1,000 mg of calcium and 1,000 IU of vitamin D.
- Antioxidant formula: Look for an antioxidant supplement that contains ingredients found in the list on pages 152–153.

Most health food stores now feature supplement sections, and their staff can help you differentiate among various brands and products. Your local pharmacy will stock many of these, and any national brand will do. Or you can ask for recommendations from people in your trusted circle, such as your friends, family members, or even your physician.

Remember: *Healthy, hydrated cells are the key to ageless skin and a healthy body.*

Step 3: Move More to Maximize Cellular Water through Muscle

For people already engaged in regular exercise, moving more is not such a big deal. Motivating people to be more physical when they are used to a sedentary life, however, is challenging. In fact, it can *backfire*; new research suggests telling people to exercise and extolling its virtues alongside the vices of fat can inspire someone to eat more junk and avoid exercise entirely! (The reason being that the attempt to motivate someone to move when he or she is, say, sitting on the couch eating is encouraging that person to do *something*, and because food is available, eating becomes the thing to do.)

The secret is to exercise for pleasure. You should be driven less by exercise's health and body-sculpting rewards (and its hydrating effects—see chapter 6) than by how working out makes you *feel*. See if you can choose one activity this week (or next, if starting with your diet is enough) and plan to do more of that activity. This doesn't have to be a Herculean effort. Go easy at the start and just get your circulation moving faster and for longer and longer periods of time. Schedule daily walks or call a friend in the morning and ask, "What can we do today?" Do jumping jacks and stretch in front of the television rather than lying on the couch. Plan a Saturday night dancing with your spouse or a group of friends. If you don't belong to a gym, ask a coworker who is a member to take you to her favorite group exercise class. You never know, you just might fall in love with it.

Remember: Take pleasure in every minor success.

Step 4: Practice Self-Discovery and Check Your Attitude

You already know in your heart that taking care of yourself sets the tone of your life and health. Some of us walk around with a keen sense of who we are and what we want to become in life, whereas others feel less certain and continually struggle to find those answers. No matter where you are in your own emotional journey, it helps to examine your attitude and perspectives. This is important in addressing the emotional-care aspect of Inclusive Health. How can this be done?

Okay, so maybe you're not a poet, a blogger, or someone who keeps a journal. I'm not asking you to be any of those, but you'd be surprised by what taking just three to five minutes at the end or start of your day to evaluate how you feel and what you're thinking at a subconscious level can do to your sense of well-being, peace of mind, and even your capacity to dream big, set realistic goals for the future, and realize optimal wellness. Self-care begins with self-discovery. And committing your thoughts and ideas to paper can make a huge difference. It affords you a record from which to look back in the future and simultaneously offers accountability. It also gives us a chance to adjust our attitudes if need be and set a new course that moves us closer to where we want to be. Find a comfortable spot (or just do this exercise while sitting in bed) and consider playing some relaxing music.

So few of us take the time anymore during our days serving and caring for others to turn the volume down on everyone and everything else and just think in our own creative space and quietude. Following are some questions to help get you started if you don't know what to write about:

1. What would you do if you knew you could not fail?
2. What job or hobby would you like to try?
3. What's the one thing you hope to accomplish in your lifetime that you haven't yet?
4. What was your childhood ambition? What is your adult ambition?
5. What are the top three things on your to-do list (that don't entail regular chores and the usual aspects of daily life)?
6. What in life is causing you a great deal of stress and anxiety? How can you begin to remedy that one step at a time?
7. What are you most proud of?

You may find it helpful to keep more than one journal. Have one that you use to write down the more mundane tasks you need to get gone, such as picking up clothes from the cleaners, grocery shopping, or organizing a birthday party. Have another that keeps track of your diet choices and physical activities. Yet another journal, a so-called worry journal, can be very handy for people who have a hard time getting to sleep at night as stressful thoughts intrude and steal much-needed sleep time. A worry journal by your bedside can act as a mental depository of your anxieties. Once you write them down, you close the book and tell yourself that you will deal with them tomorrow. Sometimes you'll find that the act of writing down a worry will lead to solutions that you never thought of before. And all of these exercises will subconsciously give you hope for your future.

Last but certainly not least, keep a positive-note journal that tracks all the good things you've accomplished. At the end of even the most stressful days, stop to reflect on what went right. What are you grateful for? What good things came out of the day, even if they were unplanned or unexpected? Sometimes, on the worst of days, we can just be thankful that we got through it, and soon we can embrace a whole new day with happy, promising thoughts and intentions.

Remember: Allow spontaneity in your life.

Step 5: Savor Sleep to Lock in Youth and Water

Insufficient sleep may well be the biggest health-related lifestyle problem in America. It creates a domino effect that not only raises the risk for a bevy of health challenges from cardiovascular issues to obesity, depression, and immune impairment, but also lowers the threshold for enduring stress. The vast majority of Americans—almost three-quarters of us—don't get enough high-quality sleep. This explains not just chronic exhaustion but also low cellular water content and even thicker waistlines. In chapter 8 I'll explain the role of sleep in the Water Secret and offer tips to a better night's sleep. For now, put this on your agenda, and close to the top if you can.

If you've grown accustomed to sleep aids, whether prescription or over-the-counter, see if you can wean yourself off those once you begin to implement the Water Secret in your life. Although sleeping aids do serve a purpose at certain times of one's life, they should not be used long-term, and many of them can infringe on restorative deep sleep—the kind we need to feel truly refreshed and rejuvenated the next day.

Mary T. is but one patient who typifies the typical sleep-aid abuser. She's hooked to caffeine to keep herself charged through the day, and then finds herself staying up late at night to finish housework and plan for the next busy day. Once the kids have gone to bed, it's hard not to raid the kitchen and start munching on sugary foods that keep her awake, which prevents her body from slowing down for a good night's sleep. That's usually when she logs online to take care of e-mail and surf the Internet. By the time she knows it's time for bed (because there are only six hours left to sleep), she has to pop a sleep aid, and the vicious cycle repeats itself the next day.

It took Mary just three months to end her relationship with sleep aids using the strategies I'll outline in chapter 8. She said that a lot of her reliance on the sleep aids came out of habit rather than necessity. Once she began to pay attention to the clock, however, and avoid late-night eating and Internet playing, she was able to wind her body down sooner and prepare for restful sleep. She established a new habit in getting ready for bed, and with that came replenishing sleep.

Remember: Reduce Internet isolation. Sleep better.

Step 6: Try Something New, and Work with Your Passions and Talents as Much as Possible

Remember how exciting that first day of school was back when you were entering the third or fourth grade? It's thrilling to enter a new environment, meet new people, and learn something different. Adults trying to keep up with their everyday obligations rarely give themselves permission to act like a schoolgirl or schoolboy again, but doing so can have some surprising benefits. In addition to expanding your horizons and exposing you to a new hobby or skill, trying something new can take you just far enough away from your established and routine commitments to give you the feeling that you're on vacation, that you're allowed to goof off and replenish the kid in you again that's unencumbered by the banalities of everyday life.

Think about your current hobbies or one you'd like to try, and see if you can find a club, group, or class nearby in which to participate. This can be any number of things, including cooking class, a writing class, a pottery workshop, a photo club, or a book club. And if you can't find anything attuned to your interests, then start your own club or group and invite your friends.

Not all of us can say we are 100 percent satisfied with our current job. Although it can take time, patience, and trial and error to find and flourish in a career that's deeply fulfilling and enriching, that doesn't mean you can't find a certain level of enjoyment and gratification in whatever job helps you meet your obligations now. You will continue to explore opportunities in the hopes of finding and establishing yourself in the ideal work scenario. After all, in any job there are bound to be periods of frustration, high stress, and maybe anguish. Even people who are lucky to have already found their dream job experience challenges that require them to refocus or test a new and unplanned path. Taking stock of your feelings about your work life is critical to your Inclusive Health plan. Your emotional health is a big piece to the health puzzle, constituting a third prong to overall wellness. We spend the majority of our waking days working, so it's vital that those long days are contributing to our mental and physical health—not taking it away. This is possible when we strive to align our goals and values with our talents and passions in a job that supports our livelihood, and allows us to feel appreciated and needed in the world at large.

Remember: Make trailblazing a way of life. Try something new.

Step 7: Give Back

In Step 10 I'll encourage you to plan events with friends and family—people with whom you share deep connections. Setting aside time with those who can help us relax and move away from the limelight of stress is important for our emotional and physical health. As you'll read in chapter 8, one of the triggers of Cultural Stress is isolation. Even though we have more gadgets now than ever to connect with others through phones and computers, we also have a higher number of people complaining of loneliness and feelings of disconnectedness. It seems like the more connections we make on the surface, the more we lose out on opportunities to nourish and renew those much deeper and rewarding connections in person.

Of the patients I've seen who appear to have a tremendous amount of Cultural Stress in their lives, those who don't have a solid group of friends and regular plans to visit with them are the worst off. Their Phase Angles are lower, their hydration figures are below average, and signs of aging are more visible. But sometimes it's not enough just to suggest that they spend more time with friends. They need to go a step further, and engage in an activity that rewards them not just with friendships, but also with a positive outcome that has the added benefit of affecting others. In other words, they need to give back.

Have you ever signed up to volunteer at community events? Have you ever offered your time and expertise to a local youth club or adult-education center? Have you ever joined a mentorship program that matches you with another individual who wants to learn your skills? Have you ever watched a group of volunteers cleaning up a park or beach and wished you could join them? There are dozens of ways you can give back. Though the media like to focus on how giving back is the practical way in which each one of us can have an impact in the world and effect global change, I like to think about what it gives the person who is doing the giving back: a chance to forge new friendships, to squelch feelings of isolation and stress, and to enjoy the act of making a difference that will surely make a difference on a much smaller—yes, *cellular*—level.

Remember: Explore your hidden opportunities.

Step 8: Water and Treat Your Skin

It wouldn't surprise me to learn that the vast majority of people don't keep a regular skin care routine. The consequences aren't as painful as, say, not brushing your teeth every day. But they can be very noticeable in the decline of your looks and acceleration of your physical age. The time it takes to treat your face is the same as it is to brush your teeth—about two minutes. Any drugstore can get you started. At the very least, get a gentle daily cleanser and two types of moisturizers: one with sunscreen, and a night cream without. Add to that an exfoliator to use a few times a week or as your skin needs it, and any special formulas you may want to include in your regimen (see chapter 7 for details). Pamper your face twice a day. Splurge on a facial or some other special treatment offered at spas a few times a year, or as often as you can.

Remember: Healthy skin is a reflection of overall wellness.

Step 9: Relax

As I mentioned above, we'll see in chapter 8 how pervasive Cultural Stress can be in our rapid-fire culture. It sounds almost cliché to say "relax" because it will "reduce stress," since this is like telling someone not to breathe (or check e-mail). Stress will always be part of our life—and our livelihood. The key is to keep certain sources of unnecessary stress at bay so they don't affect us like a charging rhino. Easier said than done, but here are some things to think about this week:

- Can you set a time each day after which you turn off your cell phone and don't respond to nonemergency calls, e-mails, text messages, and so on?
- Can you create a bedtime routine that prepares you for sleep thirty minutes prior to lights out?
- Can you make it a goal to treat yourself once a month or as often as feasible to a massage or another therapeutic treatment of your choice?
- Can you plan your days better so you're not as harried?
- Can you take a recess for some deep breathing or meditation when problems present themselves and your mind starts to race? Problems can easily swell into unmanageable-portion sizes for our consciousness and bring us down. Then they get out of control and look worse than they really are. Deep breathing or meditation will help you to gain perspective and reclaim sanity again. (See box on page 100 for a deep-breathing and meditation exercise.)
- Can you get outside more to enjoy the calming effects that only nature can provide? So few of us spend time outdoors anymore. We live and work indoors, often chained to electronics, meetings, and chores. But being outdoors and among plants and other living things can enhance feelings of health and well-being. This is partly why going for walks and hikes or sailing, skiing, cycling—doing anything in the open air—can be so invigorating. Don't forget to bring the outdoors in, too. Park a big live plant in the room where you spend the most time each day. Set up a reading chair beside a window where you can observe trees and birds.
- Can you pick just one single habit you want to change and make a commitment to making that happen? It can be an ambitious goal such as quitting smoking or a small one such as reducing your consumption of fast food or replacing butter with extra-virgin olive oil in your cooking.

I know your answer to all these questions is a resounding yes. But if not, then choose to say yes and watch what happens.

Remember: Equal parts vegetables and "vegging out" keep the doctor away.

Take a Deep Breath

Here's one of my favorite deep-breathing exercises. It can be done at any time and in any place. Try it lying down or sitting in a comfortable chair while maintaining good posture.

- Close your eyes and relax your body as much as possible. Scan your body from head to toe and let go of any tension.
- Pay attention to your breathing. With one hand on your heart and another on your belly, notice the rise and fall of each breath. If you are using the lower part of your lungs, your abdomen should be noticeably rising and falling. Your chest should not be rising nearly as much.
- Continue breathing deeply through your nose.
- After several more breaths, inhale slowly through your nose and exhale through your mouth. Keep your mouth, tongue, and jaw relaxed.
- Continue this pattern of methodical breathing as you stay relaxed, and focus on the sound and feeling of long, slow, deep breaths.

Meditation is not for everyone, but it's also not just for monks anymore. With time and patience, anyone can learn to meditate. It's like entering a deeply restful sleep while being fully awake; it's casting the human brain back to a more primitive state where we are freed of our analytical and critical selves. In this blissful state of mind, you are more aware of senses and feelings rather than negativity and stress. Here's a simple way to try it:

- Sit in a quiet and comfortable spot. Be mindful of your posture. Set a timer for five or ten minutes.
- Choose a word to repeat to yourself. Many people who meditate like to use the word "om" because it has been shown to be calming. Or you can murmur "breathe in" and "breathe out" to yourself, or count your breaths from one to ten, then repeat.
- Close your eyes and focus on your word or count. When thoughts intrude, gently bring your attention back to the word or count.
- Keep going as long as you can without falling asleep.
- When you're ready, slowly open your eyes. How do you feel?

Step 10: Celebrate

When was the last time you experienced truly gut-wrenching laughter with friends? One of my patients, Danielle, says, "Why wait for the weekend to get together with friends and celebrate?" This is akin to my own mantra, "Why have a bad day when you can have a good day?" That may sound jejune and trite, but planning to have a good day is very real. Danielle gathers her friends around the kitchen every Wednesday night for a homemade pizza. And she even does this during super-busy or particularly stressful weeks. Why? Because even though it's extra work to prepare for the meal, she finds pizza night to be better than therapy. And her friends agree. They keep coming back during their hardest weeks because they love what the night does to them: it rekindles their spirits and turns the volume down on their stress levels. (They love the homemade pizza, too.)

See if you can plan more time with the people who inspire and de-stress you. And don't wait for the weekend! Regular quality time with the people dear to us can be incredibly therapeutic. Strengthening those connections in real life can be as powerful as any other strategy to boost health and well-being. When we reduce our isolation, we reduce our risk for illness, and we increase the quality of our lives.

Remember: Turn the rest of your life into the best of your life.

The Ten-Day Water Secret Meal Plans

If you are ready to commit to achieving a healthy body, the next ten days can be your starting point for living by the Water Secret in your dietary choices. I promise it won't be difficult. I'm all for delicious, tasty meals full of flavor and satisfaction. You'll start your nutrient blitz by filling your body with everything it needs. Luscious whole foods with all the proper nutrients will help your cells hold onto water; you'll see and feel results almost immediately. You'll find the recipes for ideas marked with an asterisk (*) starting on page 119.

For ideas on what to drink, see page 155. I encourage you to limit beverages that contain caffeine, refined sugars, and alcohol during these ten days. Try switching to water (sparkling mineral or still) flavored with lemon, lime, or orange wedges, unsweetened fruit juices diluted with a splash of sparkling water, unsweetened iced teas, and hot herbal and green teas. If you're accustomed to drinking coffee early in the morning and soda in the late morning or afternoon, see if you can reduce your intake by having just one cup of coffee with breakfast and then opt for tea rather than soda or energy drinks the rest of the day.

If you find that these meals don't fill you up enough, it's perfectly okay to add more in terms of portions—just be careful about what you're choosing. Opt for more fruits and vegetables first, then lean proteins and complex carbohydrates. Try adding more nut butters or avocado; to satisfy an afternoon hunger pang, try a handful of almonds, walnuts, or seeds or a serving of all-natural popcorn. I've recently found Kavli crispbread to be a delicious cracker for dipping into hummus, guacamole, or peanut butter as a quick snack. This is not supposed to be a "diet" in the traditional weight-loss realm. The ideas here are meant to show you which types of foods you should be gravitating toward and how to best combine ingredients to fulfill the promise of the Water Secret. Don't be afraid to experiment.

Feel free to mix and match these meal ideas, too; use the following days' outline of ideas as a guide rather than a strict regimen. Be mindful of any allergies that you have and seek appropriate substitutes. After the tenth day you'll have a good sense of how a typical day of eating should go, so you can then begin to make your own choices (and continue to go back to any of the following ideas that you enjoy).

Bon appétit!

Day 1

The meal plans start with my Cellular Water Secret Smoothie. Every ingredient in this antiaging power smoothie contains the key nutrients and phytochemicals to optimize the water content in the cells while also building and strengthening connective tissue. Essential amino acids to encourage the healthy formation of collagen and elastin tissue are in the soy milk. Phosphatidylcholine and lecithin maintain cell membranes. The antioxidants in the pomegranate juice, blueberries, and goji berries protect against free radical damage to cell walls and connective tissue. Essential fatty acids in the flaxseed lock moisture into the cell. Anti-inflammatory compounds in some of the ingredients in this smoothie help soothe skin irritation. And most importantly, the nutritional benefits of this smoothie can help increase the water content of your cells, reduce wrinkles, and increase skin elasticity.

Breakfast

Cellular Water Secret Smoothie*

Whole-grain waffle topped with ½ cup unsweetened applesauce, sprinkle of cinnamon, and 1 teaspoon chopped walnuts

Try Kashi GOLEAN waffles, found in the frozen-foods section, or Arrowhead Mills waffle mix.

Midmorning Snack

1 cup vegetable juice of choice

Carrot and celery sticks (as many as desired)

Lunch

Chicken Vegetable Soup*

Veggie Sandwich on Whole-Wheat Pita* (chicken or salmon optional)

1 medium orange or any fruit of your choice

Midafternoon Snack

1 medium apple

2 cups air-popped popcorn

Dinner

2 cups or more as desired vegetable salad with dressing of your choice*

1 cup cooked whole wheat pasta topped with 1 cup steamed mixed vegetables (broccoli and cauliflower florets, carrot and zucchini slices) and 2 ounces cooked skinless white meat chicken (cut into cubes), or ½ cup baked and cubed tofu, covered with ½ cup marinara sauce

Dessert

½ cup fresh or unsweetened frozen strawberries

Tip of the day: Vegetable juice drinks are a great way to get more vegetables in the diet. The preferable way is to get them from vegetables. However, including vegetable juices is also beneficial and can be a concentrated source of nutrients and phytochemicals that protect and nourish the cells, promoting their hydration.

Day 2

Breakfast

½ medium grapefruit

½ cup oatmeal with cinnamon and raisins or dried goji berries with fat-free milk or soy milk

Try McCann's Quick Cooking Irish Oatmeal or Kashi Heart to Heart Oatmeal

Midmorning Snack

1 medium apple cut into slices

6 raw almonds

Lunch

2 cups or more vegetable salad with 2 tablespoons dressing of your choice

1 cup minestrone soup (buy an organic, low-sodium variety)

2–5 low-fat whole-grain crackers

1 piece fresh fruit of choice

Midafternoon Snack

2 tablespoons dried goji berries or raisins

4 walnuts

Dinner

Grilled wild fish of your choice with lemon and dill

½ cup steamed brown rice

Roasted Greens*

Dessert

Fresh fruit platter (a wide variety of colorful fruits) with ½ cup Greek-style or soy yogurt

Greek-style yogurt is loaded with protein and is very low in sugar and calories. Try Fage 0 percent or 2 percent instead of the 260-calorie-a-cup whole-milk yogurt.

Tip of the day: Oatmeal is one of the best whole grains to include in a heart-healthy diet. It includes soluble fiber to help lower cholesterol, and this fiber also helps to keep blood sugar under control. Oats also are a natural source of antioxidants.

Broccoli is high in vitamin A (beta-carotene) and vitamin C, two important antioxidants to protect our cells from damage. The vitamin A and various phytochemicals, such as isothiocyanates, indoles, and bioflavonoids, in broccoli may help prevent cancer. Broccoli also is a good source of calcium.

Day 3

Breakfast

2 poached eggs or ½ cup steamed tofu seasoned with soy sauce or Bragg's Liquid Aminos

1 slice whole-wheat toast with almond butter and strawberry jam

Bragg's Liquid Aminos is a substitute for soy sauce and can be found at health food stores and Whole Foods markets. It's nonfermented and doesn't contain added salt, but it tastes the same.

Midmorning Snack

1 cup or more as desired raw vegetables of choice

2 Scandinavian-type whole-grain rye crackers

Try Rye-Crisp or Wasa high-fiber crackers

Lunch

2 cups or more as desired tossed green salad with 2 tablespoons dressing of your choice

1 cup Vegetarian Split Pea with Barley Soup*

1 whole grain roll

½ cup fresh or frozen unsweetened blueberries

If you buy prepared salad dressing, opt for brands that are all-natural. Avoid dressings that are high in sugar and artificial ingredients such as high-fructose corn syrup, modified corn starch, and monosodium glutamate. You do not need to opt for fat-free varieties, but be careful about portions. Use a measuring spoon to drizzle a single serving of dressing over a salad.

Midafternoon Snack

Veggie Antioxidant Juice Smoothie*

2–5 whole-grain crackers

Dinner

2 cups or more as desired mixed green salad with 2 tablespoons Flax-Goji Golden Citrus Dressing*

4 ounces grilled salmon with lemon juice or 4 ounces grilled vegetarian soy chicken

½ cup brown rice pilaf

1 cup or more as desired steamed fresh broccoli

Dessert

Frozen banana slices (from one medium-ripe banana) lightly sprinkled with unsweetened cocoa powder and cinnamon

Tip of the day: Instead of using butter or margarine on your toast in the morning for breakfast, use 100 percent whole-fruit jam and spreads. These jams contain no added sugar, and when made from berries such as blueberries also add important antioxidants to the diet.

Low in saturated fat and rich in heart-healthy monounsaturated fats and flavor, olive oil is an excellent vegetable oil to have in your kitchen. Extra-virgin olive oil is considered the finest olive oil. Extra-virgin olive oil is made without heat or solvents, from the first pressing of the olives. It is the most flavorful of the different types of olive oil, and most importantly, extra-virgin olive oil contains the highest amount of healthy polyphenol antioxidants of all olive oils. When preparing foods I recommend using extra-virgin olive oil as the best type of olive oil.

Day 4

Remember, the meal plans are not low-carb diet plans. In fact, there are plenty of healthy carbs in these plans that provide the body the nutrients and energy it needs for optimal health. In these diet plans we emphasize eating only whole grains, not the refined, processed grains most Americans eat too much of that turn quickly into sugar. Whole grains are complex carbohydrates and provide important fiber as well as essential nutrients such as B vitamins.

Breakfast

Cellular Water Secret Smoothie*

½ large grapefruit

2 slices whole-grain toast with fruit jam

Midmorning Snack

1 cup red or purple grapes

1 hard-boiled egg or 1 cup soy, skim, or 1 percent milk

Lunch

2 cups or more as desired tossed green salad with 2 tablespoons dressing of your choice

1 cup Chicken Vegetable Soup* or Vegetarian Split Pea with Barley Soup*

2–4 Scandinavian-type whole-grain rye crackers or Kavli crispbread

Midafternoon Snack

1 cup or more raw vegetables with optional salad dressing for dip

6 raw almonds

Dinner

2 cups or more as desired vegetable salad with 2 tablespoons dressing

Steamed Vegetables with Marinara Sauce*

Medium baked potato brushed with 1 teaspoon flaxseed oil and sprinkled with herbal seasoning

Dessert

½ cup plain yogurt or soy yogurt topped with ½ cup fresh or unsweetened frozen strawberry slices

Tip of the day: While generally I recommend eating as many of your fruits and vegetables raw and uncooked as possible, there are ways of preparing your vegetables to minimize their nutrient loss during food preparation. One of the best and nutritional ways to cook vegetables is to steam them. You steam when you place your vegetables on a rack or in a basket above boiling water. The food should not touch the water, because nutrients can be lost in the water. Lightly steamed vegetables are excellent, as they retain many of the important nutrients found in their uncooked state.

Microwaving vegetables is a quick and nutritional way to cook them with little or no water. You also can minimize the fat in this type of food preparation. Make sure not to overcook your vegetables when using the microwave; cook them for only short periods of time.

Stir-frying with small amounts of olive or canola oil and water or vegetable broth is another nutritious way to prepare your vegetables. When stir-frying, be sure to cook them until just tender and use as little oil or liquid as possible to retain nutrients.

Day 5

Breakfast

1 cup vegetable juice cocktail

Sumptuous Veggie Scramble* with a whole-wheat English muffin

1 medium orange or other fruit of your choice

Midafternoon Snack

1 cup or more as desired raw vegetables of choice with optional dressing as a dip

Lunch

2 cups or more as desired tossed green salad with 2 tablespoons dressing

Roasted turkey sandwich on whole-grain bread with Dijon mustard, tomatoes, and avocado

Fresh medium apple

Midafternoon Snack

½ or 1 whole raw bell pepper sliced and dipped in hummus (2 tablespoons of hummus)

Dinner

Grilled chicken breast with sauce of your choice or a 4-ounce serving of any cold-water fish such as salmon or black cod. (My favorite way to season a good fish is with a sprinkle of sumac or a marinade consisting of one tablespoon olive oil, one tablespoon lemon juice, one teaspoon of Dijon mustard, and one teaspoon of crushed ginger—shake it all up and pour the glaze over the fish prior to cooking.)

1 cup steamed brown rice

Roasted Greens*

Dessert

1 cup fresh fruit salad

Tip of the day: Getting your essential amino acids from healthy protein foods is important for the formation of collagen and elastin tissue. The Pitcher of Health (described in chapter 5) includes protein selections that are best for building healthy cells by providing the body with the essential amino acids. Fish and skinless white-meat poultry are better choices of protein. Among fish, salmon and black cod are an ideal choice because they are a rich source of omega-3 fatty acids, the type of fat essential to have healthy, hydrated cells. Studies also suggest that omega-3 fatty acids play a role in protecting against cardiovascular disease and enhancing brain function. (For a list of fish ideas, see pages 148–149.)

Try to get protein from plant sources as well. By doing so you are getting your amino acids from the original sources of amino acids: plants. There are many health benefits to eating vegetable protein foods as opposed to animal sources of protein. Vegetable proteins contain no cholesterol or saturated fat and in many cases also provide a good source of dietary fiber.

Day 6

Avocados are known for their high fat content; however, they contain healthy monounsaturated fat and contain no cholesterol, so they're a healthy choice that not only enhances your overall condition but also makes your skin glow. Avocados contain lutein, a phytochemical with important antioxidant properties.

Breakfast

½ grapefruit

1 multigrain pancake topped with a handful of fresh blueberries.

Try Arrowhead Mills multigrain pancake mix.

Midmorning Snack

Cellular Water Secret Smoothie*

Lunch

2 cups or more as desired tossed green salad with 2 tablespoons dressing of your choice

Avocado-vegetable sandwich on whole-grain bread

1 medium orange or other fruit of your choice

Midafternoon Snack

6 almonds

Carrot sticks, as many as desired

Dinner

Tomato slices, as many as desired, with vinaigrette dressing

5-ounce grilled salmon steak or grilled vegetarian soy burger patty

Steamed asparagus, as much as desired, flavored with lemon juice

Whole-wheat roll served lightly brushed with olive oil; opt for wild salmon or try a Boca veggieburger

Dessert

1 cup fresh fruit salad

Tip of the day: In the Pitcher of Health only whole grains are listed. Refined-grain foods and products are not part of the meal plan. This is because when you refine grains you take away so much of their good nutritional value. Whole grains include grains such as wheat, corn, rye, oats, barley, quinoa, and spelt, when these grains are eaten in their "whole" form. Whole grains even include popcorn! Eating whole grains has been shown to reduce the risks of heart disease, stroke, cancer, diabetes, and obesity. In their natural state, whole grains are the entire seed of a plant. This seed, which is called the kernel, is made up of the bran, the germ, and the endosperm. The bran contains important antioxidants, B vitamins, and fiber. The germ is the embryo; if fertilized by pollen, it will sprout into a new plant. It contains many B vitamins, protein, minerals, and healthy fats. An example is that wheat germ is a good source of vitamin E. The endosperm part of the grain contains starchy or complex carbohydrates and proteins. Eating whole grains (and avoiding refined grains) is an important part of the Water Secret diet.

Day 7

Breakfast

Cellular Water Secret Smoothie*

½ cup oatmeal with cinnamon and fat-free milk or soy milk

½ medium or 1 cup cubed cantaloupe

Midmorning Snack

1 medium orange

4 raw walnuts

Lunch

2 cups or more as desired vegetable salad with 2 tablespoons dressing

1 cup lentil soup

1 whole-wheat roll

1 medium apple

Midafternoon Snack

1 cup or more as desired raw vegetables with optional dressing for dip

1 cup fat-free or 1 percent milk, or soy milk, or ½ cup lowfat cottage cheese

Dinner

2 cups or more as desired tossed green salad with dressing

Asian Stir-Fry Vegetables with Skinless Chicken or Tofu*

⅓ cup cooked brown rice

Dessert

½ cup fresh or frozen unsweetened blueberries

Day 8

Flax-Goji Golden Citrus Dressing is a flavorful dressing and is great on salads and raw veggies. It provides omega-3 fatty acids (from flaxseed oil), antioxidants (from goji berries and lemon and orange juices), and B vitamins (from the nutritional yeast flakes). All these ingredients help provide your body with nutrition essentials to build healthy cells.

Breakfast

1½ cups mixed fresh fruit bowl topped with fruit-flavored yogurt or soy yogurt and sprinkle of chopped walnuts

Midmorning Snack

1 cup tomato juice cocktail with a squeeze of lemon or lime juice

Carrot and celery sticks, as much as desired

Lunch

2 cups or more as desired tossed green salad with 2 tablespoons Flax-Goji Golden Citrus Dressing*

Deli sandwich of your choice (my favorite is hummus spread on two slices of whole-grain pita bread, with tomato and cucumber slices placed in between with some alfalfa sprouts or pumpkin seeds for an added crunch)

1 cup steamed broccoli seasoned with lemon juice and minced

garlic

Midafternoon Snack

1 sliced bell pepper; dip the slices into 2 tablespoons Hummus*

Dinner

Chicken and Black Bean Burrito*

Dinner Party Secret Salad*

Dessert

⅓ medium cantaloupe

Tip of the day: Flaxseeds are an ancient food that was used by Hippocrates, "the Father of Medicine," for improving the health of his patients. Today, modern nutrition researchers have identified several substances in flaxseed that have health benefits. These include lignans, fiber, and omega-3 fatty acids. Lignans are phytoestrogens that may play a role in preventing hormonally related cancers of the breast and endometrium (the lining of the uterus). Flaxseed also is a good source of cholesterol-lowering soluble fiber. Flaxseed is rich in alpha-linolenic acid, which is an essential fatty acid and an omega-3 fatty acid. The essential fatty acids in flaxseed help lock moisture in the cells and are a key nutritional component of the Water Secret diet.

Walnuts are another excellent plant source of omega-3 fatty acids. Some nutritionists believe that walnuts will become "the next fish oil" as a popular omega-3 fat source. In addition to their healthy fats, they are an excellent source of phosphorus, zinc, copper, and thiamin. In addition to eating them plain, they can easily be added to salads and sprinkled or incorporated in their ground form in many recipes.

Almonds also are a great healthy nut to include regularly in your diet. They contain healthy monounsaturated fats, an acceptable fat for the Water Secret menu plane. Try almond butter as an alternative to peanut butter. Nutritionally almonds have more calcium than any other nut and are excellent source of iron, riboflavin, and vitamin E. Remember, almonds contain a significant amount of fat (although healthy fat) and calories. So eat them in moderation, in quantities to provide your body with what it needs for healthy fat without weight gain.

Day 9

When eating fresh raw fruits such as in the fresh fruit platter, choose the brightest colors possible and a variety of different-color fruits. "Eat a rainbow" of colors every day. The more colorful and the more variety of colors you eat, the more variety of nutrients, the more important phytochemicals such as antioxidants will be provided to your body for increased cellular nutrition and protection against free-radical damage.

Breakfast

1 poached egg or ½ cup Steamed Tofu* seasoned with soy sauce or Bragg Liquid Aminos

2 slices multigrain toast with sugar-free fruit jam

½ cup fresh or frozen unsweetened strawberries

Midmorning Snack

1 medium apple

4 macadamia nuts

Lunch

Nonfat or low-fat cottage cheese or ½ cup fat-free, sugar-free plain yogurt or soy yogurt

Midafternoon Snack

Smoothie of your choice

Carrot and celery sticks, as many as desired

Dinner

2 or more cups as desired vegetable salad with dressing or your choice

4 ounces grilled fish of your choice or grilled tofu with Tomato Salsa*

⅓ cup cooked brown rice pilaf

Steamed asparagus flavored with lemon juice

Dessert

Smoothie of your choice

Tip of the day: Oranges and other citrus fruits are high in the antioxidants, vitamin C, and bioflavonoids. These antioxidants prevent oxidation and damage to our cells by free radicals. Whole oranges (but not orange juice) also are good sources of fiber. I recommend eating oranges in their whole form, as opposed to just getting your oranges from orange juice.

In the Pitcher of Health, nonfat and low-fat yogurt are listed as protein foods. Yogurt also is a good source of calcium and riboflavin. It is also a great source for "friendly" bacteria that aid in digestion and help maintain the health of our intestines. In North America, the two most common friendly bacteria strains used to make yogurt are *Streptococcus thermophilus* and *Lactobacillus bulgaricus*. These two types of friendly bacteria change the milk's sugar (called lactose) into lactic acid, which is responsible for yogurt's tangy taste. If you don't eat dairy products, soy yogurt is widely available and is an excellent alternative.

Day 10

When preparing a mixed green salad, try to incorporate as much variety of green, leafy vegetables as you can. Be adventurous: try new types of greens and lettuces in your salads. Experiment. Try bitter greens – they are important health supporters. As a general rule, the darker the greens, the better the nutrition. The more variety you can use, the more increased nutrition and the more new flavors you can enjoy.

Breakfast

½ grapefruit

½ cup low-fat granola or 1 cup whole-grain cereal served with fat-free or 1 percent milk, or soy milk

1 slice whole-wheat bread with fruit jam

Midmorning Snack

1 medium orange

4 walnuts

Lunch

2 cups or more as desired mixed green garden salad with dressing of your choice

Deli sandwich of your choice on whole-wheat bread

1 medium apple slices

Midafternoon Snack

Smoothie of your choice

Dinner

1 cup or more as desired raw vegetables with dressing of your choice

1 cup Vegetarian Chili*

1 medium baked potato seasoned with shaved parmeggiano reggiano or low-fat sour cream

Dessert

1 cup cubed fresh melon

Tip of the day: Kale is one of the best sources of vitamin K (providing more than 1,300 percent of the daily value, which refers to your daily recommended intake) and vitamin A (providing 3,540 percent of the daily value) for a one-cup serving, which has only 36 calories. This superfood is an excellent source of vitamin C and manganese and is a good source of fiber and copper. Kale contains the highest amount of calcium among vegetables.

Eating kale and other green, leafy vegetables is important to provide nutrients and protective factors for cell health leading to increased hydration of cells. Note that you needn't worry about "overdosing" on nutrients or vitamins when you ingest them as part of food. You're not likely to suffer from toxic levels of vitamin K, for example, from eating too much kale.

Checking In

After following the diet and menu plan for ten days or more, you should begin to see improvements in your health and well-being as well as your physical appearance. You may lose some weight if you were overweight when you started. You also may realize some improvements in your blood pressure and cholesterol, especially if you previously had high blood pressure and high cholesterol. Because of the increased fiber in the diet, you may notice increased regularity. You may experience a higher level of energy and improved sleep. Furthermore, you may see an improvement in the appearance of your skin and even notice a more youthful glow.

If you experience any of these changes, this could very well be attributed to having optimized your intracellular water and by strengthening the connective tissue. If I were to examine you in my laboratory, I would probably also see an increase in your Phase Angle, which would indicate an increase in the health and vitality of your cells. This change is largely due to the critical nutritional cellular support you received from the key nutrients (e.g., amino acids, essential fatty acids, antioxidants, phytochemicals, vitamins, and minerals) in the foods in this diet and menu plan as well as from the nutritional supplements you may have been taking.

These meal plans do not constitute just another diet that you follow for only a specified time. They are nutritional lifestyle guides you should continue to follow for the rest of your life. This is vital to keep your body, right from the cellular level, functioning at its optimal level. The meals and recipes in these meal plans are examples of the type of foods and diet needed to achieve optimal health and well-being. I encourage you to continue on this nutritional path of healthy eating and nutritional supplementation, which is critical to your ongoing success in following the Water Secret plan. By doing so you will reap the benefits of a long and healthy life. Chapter 5 will reveal my Water Pitcher of Health and show you how to create your own menu attuned to your personal preferences.

Recipes

Cellular Water Secret Smoothie

½ cup pomegranate juice (unsweetened)
½ cup soy, low-fat, or nonfat milk
½ cup blueberries (fresh or unsweetened frozen)
1 tablespoon lecithin granules
1 tablespoon ground flaxseed
2 tablespoons dried goji berries
3 to 4 ice cubes or crushed ice (optional)
Stevia extract (optional) to taste

Combine all ingredients in a blender until smooth.

Tropical Protein Smoothie

1 cup pineapple juice
½ banana
1 scoop soy protein isolate powder
Crushed ice

Combine all ingredients in a blender until smooth.

Tip: For more energy add 2 tablespoons dried goji berries, flaxseed, or pumpkin seeds.

Veggie Antioxidant Juice Smoothie

¾ cup fresh carrot juice
¼ cup fresh natural unfiltered apple juice

2 dark green lettuce leaves
1 scoop soy protein isolate powder
2 spinach leaves
¼ cup chopped fresh broccoli
2 sprigs parsley
½ teaspoon diced ginger root

Combine all ingredients in a blender and liquefy.

Sumptuous Veggie Scramble

1 tablespoon lentils (cooked and ready to go)
1 to 2 eggs
Small drizzle of olive oil, or use a cooking spray
1 to 2 cups raw vegetables (try scooping from a bag of mixed, precut veggies)

Add lentils to one or two scrambled raw eggs in a bowl.

Drizzle olive oil in skillet or use an olive oil cooking spray to coat bottom. Cook raw vegetables until slightly soft.

Pour egg mixture on top of veggies, combine all ingredients, and cook until egg is done.

Chicken Vegetable Soup

2 cups vegetable broth
1 cup fresh or frozen corn kernels
1 celery stalk, diced
1 small carrot, diced
1 small onion, diced
1 cup cooked skinless, boneless chicken breast, diced or shredded
½ cup tomatoes, diced

2 tablespoons fresh parsley, finely chopped
Spices of your choice to taste

In a saucepan, combine the vegetable broth, corn, celery, carrot, and onion. Bring to a boil.

Reduce the heat, cover, and simmer for 25–30 minutes or until the vegetables are tender.

Stir in the chicken, tomatoes, parsley, and salt and pepper. Heat thoroughly.

Makes 6 servings.

Vegetarian Split Pea with Barley Soup

1 cup split peas, rinsed and drained
2 carrots, diced
2 stalks celery, diced
1 medium onion, minced
6 cups water or vegetable broth
¼ cup barley, rinsed and drained
1 bay leaf
¾ teaspoon sea salt
⅛ teaspoon white pepper
⅛ teaspoon dried parsley
⅛ teaspoon dried thyme
1 clove garlic, minced
½ tablespoon lemon juice
1 tablespoon extra-virgin olive oil
Chopped scallions, for garnish

In a large soup pot, combine the split peas, carrots, celery, onions, and water or broth. Bring to a boil. Stir in the barley, bay leaf, sea salt, pepper, parsley, thyme, garlic, lemon juice, and olive oil. Reduce the heat and simmer, partly covered, for 1½–2 hours.

Occasionally stir as needed. Add additional salt and pepper to taste if desired.

When the soup has become thick, turn off the heat. Cover and let it sit for 15 minutes. Discard the bay leaf. Stir. Garnish with chopped scallions.

Makes 6 servings.

Flax-Goji Golden Citrus Dressing

½ cup flaxseed oil
½ cup water
¼ cup fresh lemon juice
¼ cup fresh orange juice
¼ cup dried goji berries (or dried cranberries)
3 tablespoons nutritional yeast flakes
2 tablespoons Bragg Liquid Aminos or tamari soy sauce
1 tablespoon apple cider vinegar

Combine all the ingredients in a blender and blend until smooth. Store dressing in a well-sealed jar in a refrigerator for up to two weeks.

Makes 2 cups.

Olive Oil and Lemon Juice Dressing

3 tablespoons extra-virgin olive oil
1 tablespoon fresh lemon juice
½ small clove garlic, finely minced
1 teaspoon Dijon mustard

In a small bowl, mix all the ingredients vigorously with a wire whisk.

Makes about ¼ cup, enough for 4 salads.

Olive Oil and Red Wine Vinegar Dressing

4 tablespoons extra-virgin olive oil
½ cup red wine vinegar
3 cloves fresh garlic, minced
⅛ teaspoon dried oregano
⅛ teaspoon dried thyme

Place all the ingredients in a glass container with a lid. Cover and shake vigorously.

Makes ¾ cup.

Balsamic Vinaigrette Dressing

½ cup extra-virgin olive oil
¼ cup good balsamic vinegar
Chopped garlic (about 4 cloves)
Chopped shallots (about 1 tablespoon)
1 tablespoon Dijon mustard
½ tablespoon light soy sauce
½ tablespoon honey
Rosemary (fresh or dried)
Fresh lemon juice
Pepper to taste

Combine all ingredients together *except* for the oil. Then drizzle the oil slowly into mixture as you whisk it.

Serves approximately 6.

Dinner Party Secret Salad

2–4 bags organic mixed baby greens (depending on how many people you're serving)

6–10 green onions (chopped)

Medjool dates (pitted, diced; figure 1–2 dates per person)

1 bunch cilantro (fresh, chopped)

1 bunch Italian parsley (fresh, chopped)

¼ cup rosemary (fresh leaves)

¾ to 1 can garbanzo beans

½ cup nuts (chopped, any kind or combo, such as walnuts, almonds, pecans—try roasting raw versions in oven for 7 minutes at 350° degrees).

¼ cup sunflower seeds (raw)

½ cup cheese crumbles (Gorgonzola, feta, or goat)

1 avocado, diced

The juice from 1 lemon and/or an orange

Combine ingredients in large salad bowl. Drizzle with balsamic vinaigrette.

Serves approximately 6 to 8.

Veggie Sandwich on Whole-Wheat Pita

You can add 3 ounces of cooked, cubed chicken breast or cooked, cubed salmon to the sandwich.

Tomato, ½ inch diced

Red onion, ½ inch diced

Black olives, chopped

Whole-wheat pita, cut in half to form two pockets

2 lettuce leaves

¼ cup hummus

Mix together the tomato, onion, and olives

Place a lettuce leaf in each pocket. Stuff the pockets with the vegetables and hummus, and chicken or salmon if desired.

Makes 1 serving.

Steamed Vegetables with Marinara Sauce

- 2 cups broccoli florets
- 2 cups cauliflower florets
- 2 medium carrots, diagonally cut
- 1 cup string beans, diagonally cut
- 2 medium zucchini, cut into ¼ inch rounds
- 2 medium green, red, or yellow bell peppers (or a combination), cut into 1-inch strips
- 1½ cups low-fat marinara sauce, heated

In a pot of boiling water, lightly steam the vegetables in a box steamer basket until they are cooked but still crunchy.

Arrange the vegetables on a platter. Top with low-fat marinara sauce.

Makes 4 servings.

Asian Stir-Fry Vegetables with Skinless Chicken or Tofu

Vegetable Stir Fry

- 1½ tablespoons soy sauce or Bragg Liquid Aminos
- ¼ cup vegetable broth or water
- 2 teaspoons canola oil
- 2 teaspoons minced garlic
- 1 teaspoons minced fresh ginger
- 1 large carrot, diagonally sliced in small strips

1 cup celery, diagonally sliced in small pieces

1 cup snow peas, stems and strings removed

2 medium red bell peppers cut into 1-inch strips

1 cup scallions, diagonally sliced (including green tops)

Combine the soy sauce or Bragg Liquid Aminos, vegetable broth or water, and canola oil.

Heat a nonstick wok or skillet over high heat and add the soy sauce mixture. Add the garlic, ginger, carrot, celery, snow peas, peppers, and scallions. Stir constantly while cooking over high heat for about 2 minutes. Add small amounts of additional water if needed. The vegetables should be tender and crisp.

Add chicken or tofu following the recipes below. Cook until desired temperature and texture. Serve with brown rice.

Makes 4 servings.

Prepared with Chicken

2 teaspoons tamari soy sauce or Bragg Liquid Aminos

2 teaspoons rice vinegar

½ teaspoon minced fresh ginger

½ teaspoon minced garlic

2 tablespoons vegetable broth

4 cooked boneless, skinless chicken breast halves, fat trimmed and cut into ½-inch strips

In a bowl, combine the tamari or Bragg Liquid Aminos, vinegar, ginger, garlic, and vegetable broth.

Add the chicken pieces and toss together. Cover the bowl and refrigerate for about ½ hour.

Add the chicken mixture to the wok or stir-fry.

Prepared with Tofu

¼ cup tamari soy sauce or Bragg Liquid Aminos

½ teaspoon minced fresh ginger

½ teaspoon minced garlic

1 package (14 ounces) firm tofu, well drained and cut into ½-inch cubes

Preheat the oven to 350°F. In a bowl, whisk together the soy sauce or Bragg Liquid Aminos, ginger, and garlic.

Add the tofu and gently stir to coat each cube.

Spread the tofu on an oiled baking sheet and bake for a few minutes, until the tofu is hot and golden on the outside. With a spatula, you may need to move the cubes around on the baking sheet to heat evenly while baking.

Steamed Tofu

½ cup firm tofu, cut into ½-inch cubes
4 tablespoons tamari soy sauce or Bragg Liquid Aminos
¼ teaspoon minced ginger

In a steamer, lightly steam the cubed tofu for 5 minutes.

Flavor with a mixture of soy sauce and minced ginger. Or you can use any fat-free flavorful sauce.

Chicken and Black Bean Burrito

4 ounces cooked chicken chunks
½ cup cooked black beans
¼ cup steamed fresh or frozen corn kernels, broccoli florets, and ½ inch diced carrots or other favorite vegetables
1 low-fat whole wheat tortilla
½ cup tomato salsa (see attached)

Combine the chicken, beans, and vegetables.

Place the mixture on the tortilla.

Wrap the tortilla to form a burrito.

Top with tomato salsa.

Makes 1 serving.

Vegetarian Chili

1 pound tofu, crumbled
1 tablespoon soy sauce or Bragg Liquid Aminos
1 medium onion, chopped
½ green pepper, chopped
2 cloves garlic, minced
2 tablespoons canola oil
2 cups cooked pinto beans
1 can (16 ounces) tomato sauce
1 cup vegetable stock
1 tablespoon chili powder

Stir together the tofu and soy sauce in a large bowl.

In a large pan, sauté the onion, green pepper, and garlic. Add the tofu and continue cooking until the tofu is browned.

Add the beans, tomato sauce, vegetable stock, and chili powder. Mix thoroughly. Bring to a boil.

Makes eight 1-cup servings.

Tomato Salsa

2 cups chopped tomatoes
⅓ cup chopped onions
1 4-ounce can chopped green chilies
¼ cup finely chopped fresh cilantro
2 tablespoons fresh lime juice
¼ teaspoon sea salt
Tabasco sauce to taste

Place all the ingredients in a large mixing bowl and blend thoroughly.

Makes approximately 2 cups.

Hummus

2 cups cooked or canned garbanzos (chickpeas)
⅓ cup fresh lemon juice
¼ cup tahini
2 cloves garlic
2 teaspoons extra-virgin olive oil
1 teaspoon salt
½ teaspoon onion powder
¼ cup water
Fresh parsley, chopped (for garnish)
Pinch of paprika and sumac

Combine all the ingredients in a blender and blend until very smooth. Add additional water if necessary. Garnish with chopped parsley. Sprinkle paprika and sumac as desired on top.

Makes four ½-cup servings.

Roasted Greens

1–2 pounds Brussels sprouts
1 large head broccoli
¼ cup extra-virgin olive oil
1 tablespoon chopped fresh thyme leaves or 1 teaspoon dried
1 tablespoon chopped fresh oregano leaves or 1 teaspoon dried
1 teaspoon garlic powder
½ teaspoon kosher salt
¼ teaspoon freshly ground black pepper
½ cup reduced balsamic vinegar

Heat the oven to 425 degrees F.

In bowl, combine Brussels sprouts and florets of the broccoli. Drizzle extra-virgin olive oil over veggies to lightly coat them. Add the thyme, oregano, garlic powder, salt, and pepper. Pour contents of bowl onto roasting pan and cook for 20 minutes. Shake the contents and cook for another 20–25 minutes until the veggies are browned. Drizzle vinegar over top while hot and serve.

Serves 4 to 6.

CHAPTER 5

It's Not What You Eat, It's What You *Don't* Eat

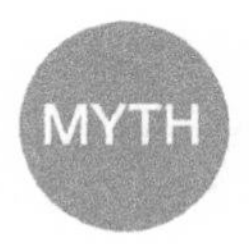

You get all the nutrition you need from "healthy," organic foods.

I'll never forget the story of Jacob, a thirty-four-year-old man who came to me for help in treating his severe acne. I first told him that I don't have acne patients—I treat patients who have acne, and there's a subtle but profound difference in that statement. A legend in my office now, Jacob's experience fits the proverbial ugly duckling tale pretty well. His painful acne aside when I first met him, Jacob didn't appear to have a strong social network and I sensed a little depression going on in him. Overweight and a bit unkempt, he admitted that he didn't like his job and found life in general to be stressful and draining. I pictured him robotically going through the motions every day and coming home to a lonely apartment and a barren kitchen devoid of nutrients his body sorely needed. No girlfriend, no roommate, and seemingly no time to engage in any activities that would support a healthy social life, let alone help him to get more active. I think he was surprised by how much time I spent with him initially, as I asked questions and encouraged him to make a few changes in his life.

His ears pricked up when I dove into the concept of the Water Secret, which I explained to him after I told him how we'd control and manage the acne. Jacob, like many others, hadn't appreciated the indelible connection between the outer skin and internal body until I described it in detail. I said you have to look beneath the surface of skin and examine the relationship of the internal aspects of the body to the health of the skin. This entails decoding not only the mechanisms of inflammation, disease, and hormones, but also the metaphorical mind and heart. It helps to picture the skin attached to every other part of the body, because it is.

Anyone can achieve radically good results in the appearance and health of the skin if physical and emotional changes are made in addition to traditional topical therapies. For Jacob, this meant shifting from a socially isolated lifestyle to a more interactive one that could help him manage stress better and meet inspiring people. I listed three things to always have on hand in the kitchen (eggs, fresh fruit, and a supplement pack), hoping that would at least get him started at paying attention to his diet. I wanted him to flush his body with nutrients to strengthen his cells' membranes and connective tissue so they could hold in the good water. I shared with him that well-hydrated cells function, heal, and renew properly, and keep the skin barrier function intact and healthy. He was surprised to learn that topical skin care products address only about 20 percent of the skin's needs. The other 80 percent have to come from proper nutrition. Even the world's most advanced, most expensive products won't give your skin a rosy glow if you're not taking good care of your internal body.

When he left that day with his acne treatment in hand, I knew I'd given him his point of entry into a new life. The acne would go away and the self-esteem he'd gain from clear skin alone would motivate him further. By the way he expressed enthusiasm for the foods and supplements I recommended he obtain (and which you'll learn about below), I had a feeling he'd follow my recommendations. More than anything, I think he enjoyed the care and personalized attention I gave him. No one else had taken a serious interest in his life lately.

About four months later, Jacob returned for a visit. I expected his acne to have cleared up, which it did, but I never could have predicted the swan that stood before me. Jacob had made major changes, all of which had started with a clear face and newly found confidence. He'd lost thirty-five pounds and found a thrilling new job that afforded him opportunities to forge friendships with like-minded people. He'd even started a relationship. I was especially moved by his crisp new wardrobe, which accented a toned body. Jacob had gone from someone who didn't seem to care how he dressed to being an aficionado of fashion.

This was an extreme makeover in the flesh, and he'd done it starting with taking better care of his skin, which then transferred to other areas of his life. He began to follow the guidelines I'd given him to put the Water Secret to the test in the kitchen, which you'll learn about shortly. He began to work out more and embrace opportunities to meet new people. He began to feel so good about himself and his appearance that he decided to live more proactively—and results were radiating from every angle of his life. Just four months previously he looked to be in his forties and now he was looking a vibrant thirty, four years *younger* than his actual age. Testing his cellular water confirmed what I could tell just by looking at him: his lab reports indicated a considerable hike in his cellular water content, and his Phase Angle had doubled from a 4 to an 8. That's a huge leap.

Jacob's story is not an anomaly. It stands out in my mind because his transformation was so incredibly visible in such a short time. His entire personality metamorphosed from a withdrawn and disheveled scruff to an uninhibited free spirit loved by his peers for his beauty and energy. And it all started with a few simple changes—treating his acne and addressing his diet—and everything else followed. For many people, especially those who don't have specific skin issues to address, the diet is the best point of entry for making a change and seeing the Water Secret in action. In fact, it's the single most influential way to repair cells and support cellular water, pure and simple. The vast majority of Jacob's transformation can be credited to the shifts he made in his diet once he felt that his acne was under control.

Let's Eat!: A New Pitcher of Health

This is not a diet book, but you will lose weight if you follow the nutritional recommendations. And you'll need to drink *less* water because you'll be getting high-quality water from the foods you eat, which will maintain strong, truly hydrated cells. Remember the goal: to put water back into the cells and keep it there. To do this the body needs to be flooded with nutrients that will strengthen cell membranes and connective tissue so they hold in the good water. It is this water that will help you to maximize and even accelerate your metabolism, sculpt stronger muscles, burn unwanted fat, and essentially live younger. In doing so, you'll give your body what it needs to heal itself, and prevent the onset of disease.

In recent years we've heard a lot of noise about the value of eating organic, whole, and "healthy" foods, and that low-fat, "good carb" diets are best. But this truth remains: you could still be missing the mark when it comes to getting all those nutrients. How many people do you know who go on traditional "diets" by restricting and eliminating certain foods, opting for "healthy" alternatives, yet still have trouble losing weight? You'll be rejoicing on the Cellular Water Secret Diet because it's not really a diet at all. You can continue to eat however and whatever you want; I am only going to ask you to follow a few secrets to healing your cells to boost their hydration. This will chiefly entail *adding*—not subtracting—foods to your life.

> Because Americans are overfed and undernourished, we tend to be overweight and underhydrated.

Most people do not realize that the skin symptoms they see in the mirror and the fatigue they feel result from nutrient deficiencies that worsen cellular dehydration. Clinical studies have shown that too little of certain nutrients can increase the risk of cancer, heart disease, osteoporosis, and premature aging. All of these then exacerbate cellular dehydration further. In my own studies, I've recorded how nutrient deficiencies result in low Phase Angles, low cellular water, and high "aging" water—the kind stuck outside cells where it doesn't belong.

About 80 percent of Americans allegedly try very hard to eat healthier, about 10 percent say they're "always successful," and yet the majority of us are overweight or obese—and chronically dehydrated. What if we've been focusing on the wrong thing? What if, instead of thinking about limiting grams of fat or which carbs to avoid, we simply ate the foods that feed our cellular membranes and encourage healthy cellular water? I think we'd see a change, and many of the problems about weight would take care of themselves. Correction: I *know* we'd see a change because I've watched hundreds of my own patients do just that.

The problem with most diets (even ones where you're simply trying to eat better regardless of weight) is that they tell you what *not* to eat, which often deprives you of critical nutrients *and* your emotional stability. Thanks to the media and recent diet books, you understand now that trans fats, refined sugar, sodium, and processed and classic fast food should be regulated in your diet. You don't need another book to tell you that. But I find that people forget to consider what they could be *missing* in their wholehearted attempts to shape up and trim down. And yes, what you could be missing probably includes healthy sugars and healthy fats. There's nothing more dehydrating than going on a nonfat, low-carb diet taken to the extreme.

It's really true that we are what we eat. If you performed a complete chemical analysis of your body, the report would list materials similar to those in foods: fat molecules, carbohydrates, protein complexes, and vitamins and minerals that help you to metabolize food and generate the energy you need to live. Think of the body as a self-maintaining factory; it is constantly regenerating itself down to every cell. Each month we renew our skin, every six weeks we have a new liver, and every three months we have new bones. To renew and rebuild these organs and tissues, we need to supply our bodies with the elements that have been lost as a result of constant use, degeneration, or aging.

Missing Ingredients

All things considered, it is important to understand that for most people, it's not what they do or don't eat or drink, it's that they are unable to keep the water they consume within their cells' membranes. And this can only be done with an adequate supply of four essential ingredients: (1) amino acids, which are the building blocks to proteins; (2) lecithin, which contains a key ingredient in cell membranes called phosphatidylcholine; (3) antioxidants; and (4) essential fatty acids.

With the appropriate amount of these nutrients, which are sorely lacking in the standard American diet, the body can maintain and build healthy, strong cell membranes that are critical to keep water from leaking out. That's exactly what the diet recommendations here will help you achieve. These nutrients come in the most delicious foods ever made on Earth. This is the undiet. You won't have to become vegan or quit cold turkey on your normal dietary habits. All I ask is that you do your best to add my recommendations to your life and watch what happens. *Feel* what happens!

Filling Up Your Daily Pitcher

There are many differences between the U.S. Department of Agriculture's food pyramid and my version, which takes the shape of a water pitcher (seen on the following page). Fundamentally, the USDA food pyramid's ultimate goal is to assist you in making healthier food and physical activity choices (the USDA version includes some exercise recommendations).

The Daily Pitcher, however, is designed to help you make the best food choices to consume the optimum level of nutrients necessary for slowing or reversing age-related cellular deterioration and improving cellular water. Highlighting fruits and vegetables above all other foods, it's a road map to maximum rejuvenation internally, externally, *and emotionally*.

The food-mood connection is powerful, and anyone who has ever overeaten or rushed to the kitchen during times of stress and anxiety knows what I mean. Mood-driven trips to the pantry or refrigerator, however, can result in reaching for foods that will drain your cells and deepen your dehydration.

The Pitcher of Health

Exercise is not included here simply because it is not a nutrient and deserves to be discussed on its own. What you also won't find in my pitcher are red meat and other high-saturated fat meat products in the protein group. It also does not contain whole-fat dairy products in the protein group, refined

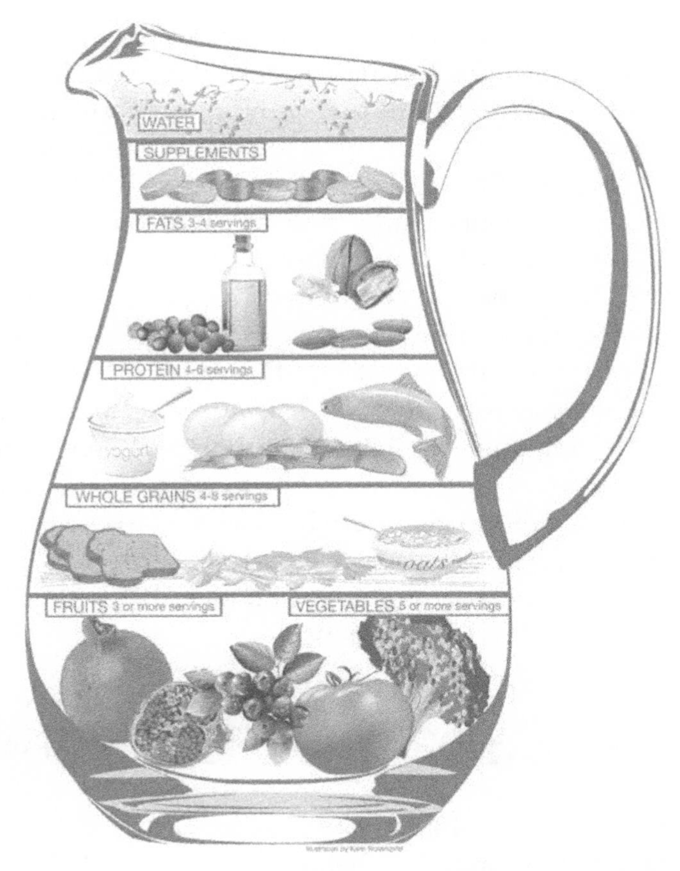

Dr. Murad's Pitcher of Health

Not All Water Is Created Equal!

Q: Why is water from a berry or a sweet potato better than plain water?

A: The water in fruits and vegetables is *structured*, meaning it's surrounded by molecules that help it get into cells easily and quickly. For this reason I encourage patients to eat—not drink—their water. Fruits and vegetables also are rich in the healing antioxidants your body needs. They also contain trace minerals and B vitamins that your body uses to metabolize carbohydrates, fat, and protein, and to synthesize DNA and new cells.

Tip: Go raw wherever possible. If you cook veggies, steam them.

grains and carbohydrates in the grain group, high-calorie refined sugars, or unhealthy fats and oils. I am not saying that you can never eat a hamburger, a hunk of Camembert, or chocolate. But as much as you can, substitute healthier alternatives. The more diligently this Daily Pitcher is followed, the more successful your results will be. I recommend using the 80/20 percent rule: eat according to this plan at least 80 percent of the time, and feel free to indulge in a few treats or favorites that aren't on here (such as a steak dinner) no more than 20 percent of the time. As I said above, approach this diet as one that teaches you how to add the nutrients you're lacking rather than eliminating anything. That slight shift in your thinking can be a powerful motivator. For more tools to following this pitcher, including a guide to what a serving would be within each food group, go to www.thewatersecret.com.

The ten-day menu plans starting on page 102 will help you put the above guidelines into action.

Whole Grains: It's Not Just about Fiber

The benefits of choosing whole grains over refined grains, which have been stripped of their outermost fibrous layer, are well documented and widely known. But what many don't realize is that the outer shell of a grain contains ingredients that the body can use to make collagen and elastin. The more collagen and elastin you create, the younger you look and feel. What's more, the skin of fruits and vegetables acts as prebiotics, nourishing a healthy balance of bacteria in the gut. This ultimately has the effect of minimizing infections and bowel problems. So the next time you're eating a whole grain, think instead about the fact that you're helping your body naturally stay young through the production of these unique "fibers" that keep your body firm and hold its shape.

Remember, collagen and elastin are fundamental to the structural network of our skin, but they go much deeper than that. Collagen in particular, which is the most abundant protein in the body, supports most tissues, gives cells structure from the outside, and is even inside certain cells. It's the main component of cartilage; ligaments; tendons; bones; and, of course, skin. It even is in the cornea and lens of the eye.

The More You Eat, the Less You'll Drink

Note how the water pitcher features water at the very top—it's not a "foundation" in the diet, as so many people think it should be. When you get your water from nutrient-dense food sources—the real foundation—you won't need to drink so much at the watering hole.

Caution on Cancer Feeders

At any given time, most people have abnormal growths, or cancer cells, in the body. Not all of these become "cancer" as we know it, though. These abnormal growths do not always show up in the standard tests until they have reached a number that's detectable and have likely started to cause problems. People who have cancerous growths in their body can often have multiple nutritional deficiencies, which is why they score so low on Phase Angle tests. An effective way to battle cancer is to starve the cancer cells by not feeding them with the foods they need to multiply. Obviously it helps to concomitantly nourish the healthy cells with what they need to thrive and prevent cancers from occurring.

So what do cancer cells love? Sugar, an acidic environment, and mucus. In addition to cutting back on refined sugar with the Cellular Water Secret Diet, ingestion of sugar substitutes such as NutraSweet, Equal, and Spoonful should be minimized. These artificial sugars are made with aspartame, which can lead to overeating. Instead, go for natural substitutes such as honey, stevia, and molasses in very small amounts.

Cancer cells thrive in the acidic environment created by meat-based diets. When you consume a diet mostly made of fresh vegetables and fruits, whole grains, seeds, nuts, and healthier source of proteins such as fish, you shift the body into an alkaline environment. The pH of a given food will change during digestion. Lemons, for example, are very acidic, but once digested, they have a very alkalizing effect. Foods usually become more acidic when cooked, which is why foods that score low on the acid test tend to be raw and "green" (think fruits and vegetables). For a list of low acid-forming foods versus high acid-forming foods, see page 143. Cancer cells also feed on mucus, which the body can produce in response to dairy products. Hormone bioactives in dairy products also can have adverse effects on skin. For these reasons, I emphasize plant sources of protein, fish, and white-meat chicken and turkey rather than beef or pork. When you do choose to eat red meat, opt for grass-fed beef, which has been shown to have lower levels of unhealthy fats and higher levels of omega-3 fatty acids. Soy and almond milk are excellent alternatives to regular milk.

Acid-Forming Foods

A Sampling of Low Acid–Forming Foods

- Apples, apricots, nectarines, bananas, berries, cantaloupe, cherries
- Beans
- Beets
- Cauliflower
- Eggplant
- Figs, dates
- Grapes
- Greens (including arugula, asparagus, avocado, beet greens, broccoli, cabbage, collards, cilantro, cucumbers, peas, lettuce, spinach, fennel, endive, zucchini)
- Olive oil
- Pumpkin
- Raw almonds, Brazil nuts, hazelnuts
- Raw seeds
- Seaweed
- Sea salt
- Soy beans, soy nuts
- Sweet potatoes, summer squash, squash
- Tangerines, mandarin oranges, mangoes
- Tomatoes

A Sampling of High Acid–Forming Foods

- Alcohol
- Artificial sweeteners
- Bacon, beef
- Candy
- Cheese
- Cocoa
- Coffee
- Fried and processed foods

(*continued*)

- Ice cream
- Jam and jelly
- Margarine
- Pudding
- Soft drinks
- Table salt
- Vegetable oil
- Vinegar
- Yeast

Nine Secrets to Keeping Your Glass (More Than Half) Full

Following are nine tips to keep in mind when shopping for and preparing food. These will maximize the repair, maintenance, and preservation of your cells so they stay strong, youthfully intact, and able to hold as much water as possible.

1. *Load up on lecithin:* Lecithin is a fatty substance in all living cells as a major component of cell membranes. It repairs tissues by helping your body build the cells with strong, watertight membranes to repair your organs and keep them fully hydrated and functioning at their highest level. It also helps to prevent gallstones and improve short-term memory. In addition to taking a daily supplement containing 2,000 to 4,000 mg of lecithin to ensure that you're getting plenty of this cell-hydrating powerhouse, choose lecithin-rich foods: eggs, non-GMO (genetically modified organisms) soy products, cauliflower, peanuts and peanut butter, oranges, potatoes, spinach, iceberg lettuce, and tomatoes. (You can find cholesterol-free powdered soy lecithin granules to add to your favorite foods and beverages. One tablespoon of soy lecithin granules has 1,725 mg of lecithin.)

Combat Hormonal Aging with Eggs

More than 70 million women today experience the effects of hormonal aging. But it doesn't start in perimenopausal years. You can experience the effects of hormonal aging *from age twenty*. The good news is that you can combat hormonal aging through diet. Estrogen is, after all, skin's best ally. I encourage all women to add eggs to their diets to preserve optimum estrogen levels naturally. If you already eat eggs, add one more to your diet per week.

2. *Add eggs and embrace other embryonic foods:* Think of complete foods or foods that have all the nutrients needed to make a full organism. In addition to eggs, these include seeds and beans, all of which are rich in embryonic material and lecithin. Many people forgo eating eggs because of cholesterol concerns; however, eggs provide nutrients that act as precursors to women's hormones and can play an important part in staving off hormonal aging. When possible, it's best to look for eggs with boosted vitamin E levels. If you are allergic to eggs, substitute with tofu or seek egg substitutes that don't contain ingredients that are problematic for you but that contain a healthy sum of egglike nutrients.

   Eggs have been taking an unfair beating lately; egg consumption has declined during the past forty years over concerns about cholesterol. But just as dietary fat is not the same as body fat, dietary cholesterol is not the same as blood cholesterol. In other words, just because you eat eggs doesn't mean you'll automatically raise your cholesterol. There's a lot more going on at the biological level. Incredibly nutrient-dense, eggs have the highest-quality protein of any food. In fact, egg protein is the standard by which other proteins are measured. The Biological Value Scale—a measurement of the efficacy with which protein is used for growth—rates eggs at nearly

94 percent, compared to a little over 74 percent for beef. Eggs also provide vitamins B2 and A, as well as iron. And to boost the value of eggs even more, last year a team of Canadian researchers showed evidence that eggs may reduce high blood pressure, and act similar to drugs used to treat high blood pressure. This came on the heels of many other studies indicating that healthy people can eat eggs without increasing their risk for heart disease.

3. *Keep the kitchen (and bathroom) stocked with antioxidants:* As detailed in the previous chapter, plants offer the best source of antioxidants—the crusaders against free radicals. Eating up antioxidants will eat up those free radicals, preventing damage and ultimately boosting hydration in cells and tissues. Choosing topical products that contain active forms of antioxidants will also help you to protect, treat, and improve your skin. In a later chapter I'll be guiding you through which ingredients to look for so you can stock your bathroom or vanity; for example, vitamin C, which protects the water-soluble portions of your cells (thus decreasing the appearance of wrinkles and enhancing the creation of collagen and elastin), can easily become deactivated by light. Only certain types of vitamin C can penetrate the skin. (So don't try to take an OJ bath or rub an orange all over you.)

   While citrus fruits and berries are the most plentiful sources of antioxidants, all fruits and vegetables provide good supplies of antioxidants. The deeper and brighter the color of the food, the more densely packed with vitamins it is. Buy the most vividly colored fruits and veggies you can find. In addition to using the list on pages 74–75 as a guide for buying fresh fruits and vegetables, following is my list of all-star antioxidants to try to keep regularly in your kitchen (or as the seasons permit):

- Blueberries, raspberries, and strawberries
- Goji berries
- Pomegranates
- Vitamin A sources: carrots, mangoes

- Vitamin C sources: kiwis, mangoes, papayas, black currants
- Vitamin E sources: vegetables oils, almonds, wheat germ, dark green leafy vegetables

If you've never tried dried goji berries, I highly recommend seeking them out at your local grocery store. They are becoming more widely available. Try them in cereal, yogurt, oatmeal, granola, smoothies, and salads.

Goji berries caught my attention ten years ago, and more recently I've discovered the benefits of durian, a fruit beloved by people in the Philippines, Thailand, and Singapore. Durian is one-stop shopping for a recipe that lives up to the Water Secret; it contains essential fatty acids and lipids, antioxidants, and anti-inflammatories—all the necessary ingredients for protecting cells from dehydration while strengthening cell membranes. The sugar compound in durian, called trehalose, stabilizes cell membranes, while the omega fatty acids help make cell membranes. Further, the sulfur in durian encourages the body to make its own antioxidants. Durian is a little harder to find in regular markets, but you can visit an Asian food store and pick up this antiaging miracle, which has both a sweet and a creamy taste. Like pomegranate, durian is highly beneficial in topical treatments, too. It provides the skin's barrier with vital lipids and good-for-you sugars that encourage cell proliferation and boost cellular water. If you cannot get past its pungent scent, look for it in topical skin treatments. (In chapter 7 I'll share which antioxidants to look for in topical ingredients. They can work wonders on skin health.)

4. *Eat three to four servings of fat a day:* Fat sounds like a four-letter word today, but the right fat in the right amount will feed your brain, your skin, and your cellular membranes like no other nutrient. Essential fatty acids (EFAs) in particular and other healthy fats keep us hydrated, supple, youthful, and beautiful. These include the unsaturated kind, such as omega-3, -6, and -9 fatty acids, flaxseed oil, extra-virgin olive oil, canola oil,

walnut oil, oil from cold-water fish, natural nut butters, seeds (ground flaxseeds, sunflower seeds, hemp seeds), and nuts (raw walnuts, almonds, cashews, Brazil nuts, and pistachios). These types of fat are full of flavor and will keep you satisfied. The menu plan in chapter 4 will show you how to get these delicious, beautifying fats into your body daily. Your body cannot make EFAs on its own, and since these are the oils that lubricate the bodies' gears, just think about what that means when you run dry.

The following is a list of top fish to buy, many of which are rich in healthy fats that you won't find in other foods to the same degree. Unless otherwise noted, aim for organic, wild-caught varieties:

- Abalone (U.S.-farmed)
- Anchovy
- Bigeye (troll- or pole-caught)
- Black cod
- Catfish (U.S.-farmed)
- Clams (farmed)
- Dungeness crab
- Halibut
- Herring
- Hoki
- Mackerel
- Mussels (farmed)
- Oysters (farmed)
- Rainbow trout (U.S.-farmed)
- Rock lobster
- Sablefish (from Alaska or British Columbia)
- Salmon (from Alaska, British Columbia, or California)
- Sardines
- Squid (from California)

Shelf Awareness

Keeping olive oil on the shelf or in the cabinet for six months can reduce its antioxidant and health benefits by up to 40 percent, according to a recent study. Don't let your storage techniques sabotage good oil. Store extra-virgin olive oil in small glass bottles (one liter maximum because the oxygen trapped in the space between the oil and top cap determines its oxidation), in a dark location, at a temperature lower than 68–77°F (20–25°C).

- Tilapia (U.S.-farmed)
- Tuna (troll- or pole-caught albacore and yellowfin)
- White sea bass

For more information about these fish and others not listed, check out the Monterey Bay Aquarium's Seafood Watch Web site at www.montereybayaquarium.org.

5. *Amplify your ALA (alpha-linoleic acid), GLA (gamma-linoleic acid), and DHA (docosahexaenoic acid):* As noted above, essential fatty acids are critical to cellular strength and water content. ALA is in the omega-3 family of fatty acids. In addition to being a great anti-inflammatory, ALA works together with antioxidants such as vitamins C and E. It's important for growth, helps to prevent cell damage, and helps the body rid itself of harmful substances that can exacerbate cellular water loss. The body also needs ALA to produce energy; it plays a crucial role in the mitochondria, the energy-producing structures of the cells, and acts as a precursor to DHA (see below). Although ALA is in vegetables, beans, fruits, flaxseed oil, canola oil, wheat germ, brewer's yeast, and walnut oil and raw walnuts, obtaining ALA from supplements is the best way to get concentrated amounts of this antioxidant (see no. 9).

Gamma-linoleic acid (GLA) is another essential fatty acid you need that comes from the omega-6 family. It feeds the brain, maintaining its structure and supporting healthy nerve function. GLA is primarily in plant-based oils. It is rarer than ALA, but can be found in seed oils such as borage, evening primrose, black currant, and hemp. As you'll learn in an upcoming chapter, this fatty acid is one of the stress-reducing nutrients largely deficient in the standard American diet. That's right: it can help you manage stress.

Docosahexaenoic acid (DHA), which can be made from ALA in the body, hails from the omega-3 fatty acid family and is the most abundant omega-3 fatty acid in the brain and the retina of the eye. A full 50 percent of the weight of your neurons' plasma membranes are composed of DHA. Low DHA levels have been associated with depression, mental decline, Alzheimer's, an increased risk for heart disease, and a higher rate of cell death among brain cells. Because of DHA's effects on brain and eye development, many prenatal vitamins for women now include DHA supplements. The best way to ensure that you're getting enough DHA is to eat plenty of fatty wild fish, and supplement with a fish oil that includes DHA. When manufactured commercially, DHA is often extracted from algae, so it's a vegetarian product.

6. *Be sure to get your Bs:* You'll find plenty of B vitamins in a variety of foods (chiefly brewer's yeast, wheat germ, whole grains, beans, dark green vegetables, low-fat and nonfat dairy, fish, eggs, and poultry), but to ensure that you get an adequate daily supply, it's best to supplement with a B complex every day that covers all eight Bs (again, see no. 9). These gems are critical to cellular metabolism and can easily be stripped from the body as a result of stress and certain medicines. Women who take the birth control pill, for example, have been shown to have low blood levels of B vitamins, which may then trigger migraines.

7. *Opt for organic and wild:* I prefer to eat organic wherever possible, but I understand that's not always a realistic option. Go organic for the following: peaches, sweet bell peppers, celery, nectarines, strawberries, cherries, pears, imported grapes, spinach, lettuce, and potatoes. When choosing chicken, go organic wherever possible. And when choosing fish, opt for wild wherever possible, too. (Again, for an updated guide to fish, go to the Monterey Bay Aquarium's Seafood Watch Web site at www.montereybayaquarium.org.)

8. *Try steviae:* There has been a lot of controversy regarding the popular sugar substitutes on the market. For those who can't do without their regular dose of sweetness, I recommend a sweet herb called stevia, which has been used worldwide for more than four hundred years without any reported side effects. Interestingly, in South America, where the herb is plentiful, the leaves have been used for centuries as a natural medicine for type 2 diabetes. It's extremely popular in Japan, where it has been used for decades. Stevia has a sweetness that is two hundred to three hundred times greater than that of sugar. New products called Truvia and PureVia have emerged on the market, and these are stevia-based sweeteners that you can now find in grocery stores. Drizzle a liquid form of stevia over low-fat Greek-style yogurt in the morning sprinkled with a handful of dried goji berries and crushed walnuts and you've got yourself a luscious Water Secret breakfast.

   And if you've got a sweet tooth and need a serious but healthy sugar fix, overripe bananas, yams, and sweet potatoes can do the trick with or without the stevia added.

9. *Fill in the final blanks with supplements:* Even the best, healthiest eater needs to take supplements today. It's simply a fact of life given our habits and stress levels (both of which can strip our bodies of nutrients). Don't panic—you won't have to swallow a cargoload of capsules or "horse pills." All of the following recommendations come in easy-to-swallow sizes and in some cases are bundled.

I like to break up my regimen to twice daily—I take a morning set with my breakfast and another with my dinner. It makes sense to do this so your body gets a constant supply of nutrients to maintain a certain balance 24-7. It's unrealistic to think that taking a single multivitamin in the morning will be useful to your body twelve hours later. But if you cannot find supplements that allow this bi-daily regimen, then once a day is okay. Avoid double-dosing up on supplements (that is, don't take a full serving of any vitamin twice a day). Although it's virtually impossible to overdose on vitamins and minerals found naturally in foods, you don't want to ingest too many vitamins in supplement form. Too much vitamin A and E, for example, is not recommended.

If you've ever had problems with digestion after taking supplements, be sure to swallow them in the middle of a meal. Don't take supplements on an empty stomach. Not all supplements are created equal. Here are the seven supplements that honor the Water Secret:

1. *Multivitamin and mineral supplement:* Select a comprehensive and balanced formula containing all the major vitamins, minerals, and trace minerals; select an iron-free formula if you are postmenopausal.
2. *Antioxidant supplement formula:* Antioxidants to look for in supplements:
   - Vitamins A, C, E
   - Alpha lipoic acid
   - Citrus bioflavonoids
   - Green tea extract
   - Grape seed extract
   - Pomegranate extract
   - Goji berry extract
   - Poria cocos
   - Milk thistle
   - N-acetyl cysteine
   - Rosemary leaf extract

- Yellow dock root
- Quercetin
- Curcumin (turmeric)
- Ginkgo biloba
- Selenium
- Coenzyme Q10

Note: While some antioxidants have a recommended daily allowance, such as vitamins A, C, and E, most do not. The general rule when recommending or using this diet is don't try to count milligrams of your antioxidant intake; instead, just try to get as many of these age-preventing all-stars in your diet as possible.

3. *High-potency B-complex supplement* providing all eight essential B vitamins: thiamine (B1), riboflavin (B2), niacin (B3), pantothenic acid (B5), pyridoxine (B6), folic acid (B9), cyanocobalamin (B12), and biotin (B7).
4. *Essential fatty acid supplement* providing omega-3 fatty acids. This may be in the form of fish oil, flaxseed oil, or ground flaxseeds added to food, or in capsule form. Vegetarians or those not eating fish or taking fish oil supplements should add a micro-algae-derived DHA supplement. Shoot for at least 500 mg of omega-3.
5. *Lecithin supplement* (2,000 mg): Lecithin can be found in capsule, powder, or granular form. Try taking 1 tablespoon of soy lecithin granules in a shake or on cereal every day (1 tablespoon = 1,725 mg of lecithin).
6. *Glucosamine supplement:* Unfortunately, your body does not produce enough of the component parts fast enough to make new connective tissue as the body routinely sustains damage and consequently loses precious water. Glucosamine is the building block for the ingredients needed to repair your connective tissues throughout your body, as well as your outermost skin layer. Unless you want to start eating unpeeled shrimp, it's best to get this nutrient in your daily supplement regimen. Take 1,200 mg of either glucosamine sulfate or glucosamine hydrochloride (HCl) every day.

7. *Calcium supplement* for bone health: Most women should take 1,000 to 1,500 mg of calcium with vitamin D daily, depending on their dietary intake of calcium. Vitamin D has gained a lot of attention in recent years due to an enormous body of research confirming its role in human health and the fact that we don't get enough of it. There's also a growing consensus that the current recommendations (400 IU per day) are far below what we really need for optimal health. If you cannot find a calcium supplement with at least 1,000 IU of vitamin D included, consider taking an additional supplement of 1,000 IU of vitamin D. Vitamin D supplements are small and easy to take with or without food. (More on this vitamin in chapter 7.)

You can find all of these formulas separately. However, some supplement formulas contain virtually all the nutrients you need in easy-to-take daily packages.

The Cellular Water Bar: What to Drink

Remember: you don't need to drink eight glasses of water a day. The stronger you adhere to the Pitcher of Health, *the less water you'll have to drink*. You'll feel and look well hydrated. You'll be able to lose the water bottle.

I'm not the first to tell you to drop or limit soda pop (diet and regular), sugar-laden fruit juices, and alcohol. If you love fruity drinks, aim for all-natural, unsweetened varieties and dilute them with sparkling water. Pomegranate and cranberry juices, for example, will be high on the antioxidant meter. Feel free to drink coffee and tea; just be careful to avoid caffeine after 2:00 P.M. or you risk having trouble getting a good night's sleep. For many, coffee is the number-one source of antioxidants daily. Researchers at the University of Scranton in Pennsylvania released a study recently that shows Americans get more of their antioxidants from coffee than any other dietary source. Both caffeinated and decaf versions appear to provide similar antioxidant levels. See if you can get more antioxidants from your fruits and veggies rather than relying on another cup of coffee.

Should you choose an alcoholic beverage, red wine is best because it naturally contains antioxidants and minerals. "Moderation" here means one six-ounce glass of wine a day for women and two for men. Have wine with food.

Fat Fact

Liquid calories present a bigger challenge to people trying to lose weight than food, according to a new study. When researchers examined the relationship between beverage consumption among adults and weight change, the greater weight loss linked to a reduction in liquid calories rather than solid foods. The results were published in the *American Journal of Clinical Nutrition* in 2009. Another study, out of the University of Texas Health Science Center in San Antonio, found that diet sodas are no body bargain, either. For every can you sip daily, your risk of becoming overweight rises by 37 percent. A 2004 study from the University of California, Berkeley, found that Americans get 7 percent of their calories from soda.

Breakfast Booster Shots

Before moving on, let me share with you my favorite two breakfasts. They are an invigorating way to start the day (yes, breakfast is still the most important meal of the day). Not only will they hold you all morning long, but they also live up to every tenet of the Water Secret.

Tasty Turkey Scramble

⅔ cup ground turkey or chicken meat (cooked and ready to go)
1 to 2 eggs
Small drizzle of olive oil or use a cooking spray
1 to 2 cups raw vegetables (try scooping from a bag of mixed, precut veggies)

Add meat to one or two scrambled raw eggs in a bowl.

Drizzle olive oil in a skillet or use an olive oil cooking spray to coat bottom. Cook raw vegetables until slightly soft.

Pour egg mixture on top of veggies, combine all ingredients, and cook until egg is done.

The Water Secret Crunchie Smoothie

½ cup blueberry juice (unsweetened)
½ cup almond milk
½ cup raspberries (fresh or unsweetened frozen)
1 tablespoon lecithin granules
½ cup pumpkin seeds
1 small banana
3 to 4 ice cubes or crushed ice (optional)
Stevia extract (optional) to taste

Place all ingredients in a blender and liquefy. The seeds will impart a delicate crunch to the smoothie.

For more recipe and meal ideas, see chapter 4.

In His Own Words

At my age, one wouldn't expect to have so many aches and pains, but I am an avid paddleboarder who trains hard throughout much of the year and participates in thirty-mile races during the summer months. I also work with my hands as a general contractor and carpenter, and enjoy working on boats for commercial fishing. So I'm constantly putting a lot of demands on my body. I spent the majority of my twenties in chronic pain, seeking minimal relief through deep-tissue massages and visiting a chiropractor. My troubles spots are my shoulders and elbows. I had to constantly ice them down and often resorted to over-the-counter pain relievers to get through my days. I never expected to have found total relief once I visited Dr. Murad, who took me through his Water Secret test. Despite my level of fitness, it was revealed that the water content in my connective tissues was abysmally low. Dr. Murad surmised that this could have been the source of all my aches and pains, and he prescribed a regimen of supplements to take that would help rebuild and rehydrate my connective tissue. Of course, I didn't believe him because I'd already been taking pretty good care of myself through my diet and took a daily multivitamin. But clearly, that wasn't enough.

Just three months after starting Dr. Murad's protocol, I noticed the change. The rock-hard tendons and ligaments that had been so tight for so long had softened, my elbows no longer locked into place, and my shoulders stayed loose and strong throughout my training season. I was sleeping better, too. Today I don't go to the chiropractor as much and I don't have to get as many massages as before just to feel a little better. It's the first time in ten years that I've felt this good. And I credit my daily regimen of supplements to recovering my connective tissues and recapturing my youth. You can't be too old or too young to rebuild and restrengthen.

—Sean R., thirty-one

CHAPTER 6

What the Fittest People Know That You Don't

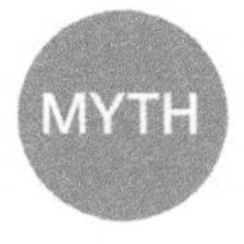

Exercise causes dehydration.

When Kate L. crossed the finish line in an October 2009 triathlon, she knew she'd clinched a personal record. The chip around her ankle clocked her at two hours, forty-nine minutes, and eighteen seconds, which meant she placed fourth in her thirty-to-thirty-five-year-old age group—the closest she'd ever come to cracking the top three competitors in a triathlon. She felt fantastic and reported back to me that it was the first time she'd ever *not* taken more than a few sips of water during the entire race. As she breezed past dozens of other competitors during the run, which was the last segment of the three-part race, she witnessed many struggling to move one foot in front of the other as they reached for water bottles strapped to their waist or accepted handouts at water stations. Granted, Kate was far behind the elite athletes who finished several minutes ahead of her, but she shared one thing in common with them: the lack of need to carry copious jugs of water and visit every water station along the course.

When I saw Kate earlier that same year, I'd taken her through understanding the Water Secret and how she could enhance her training using its concepts. The thought of not having to worry about hydration during an endurance race was particularly appealing to her, and even though she scored above average on the Phase Angle test, she believed she could do better. I sent her off with a box of supplements to take daily and ideas on incorporating the Water Secret into her life. She planned to eat more eggs, fresh fruits, and vegetables, and treat her skin daily with moisturizers and sunblock (she's a classic fair-skinned woman with sun damage from years of casual exposure in Southern California). Her training routine typically has her out in the sun for long periods of time.

While it's hard to say what exactly propelled Kate across the finish line quicker than in events past, I think it's fair to say she had an edge over others in the hydration department. In the months leading up to the race she had been bathing her body's cells in the very nutrients they needed to remain intact and water-holding. She had come to redefine what it meant to be fit. "Clearly, it's not just about strong muscles and a high aerobic capacity," she shared with me. "Looks can be deceiving. I used to be intimidated by seeing fellow competitors next to me at the start who look stunningly fit—much fitter than I. But then the race begins and everything can change pretty quickly. Suddenly I've got power from this hidden, inner fountain that affords me a source of extra strength, stamina, and agility."

Most people don't have an interest in doing a triathlon, or any sport competition, for that matter, that challenges one's overall fitness at that level. But Kate's story epitomizes what fitness should mean for everyone regardless of

Fat Fact

Fat tissue is about 10 to 20 percent water, while lean tissue (which includes muscle, bone, and water outside muscles) averages 70 to 75 percent water. Because muscle is so much denser and heavier due to the water, people who gain muscle mass and lose fat may not see the numbers tick down so fast on the scale, but their clothes become much looser!

physical conditioning and athleticism. The benefits of exercise are well documented, but if I were to ask you what some of those benefits are, chances are you'd list things such as lower heart rate, stronger cardiovascular system, higher lung capacity, weight management, and so on. The advantages of being fit are plentiful, but here's an advantage that is rarely mentioned or even considered: hydration. That's right: in the lab you'll find that people who maintain a regular physical exercise program—even just a simple, minimal routine a few times a week—have higher Phase Angles and cellular water content. They are able to stay hydrated much more easily than a sedentary person. Why? Muscle—not fat—is the ultimate compartment for cellular water. It holds much more water than fat does, which also explains why bioelectrical pulses sent through a body to measure its composition move quickly through people who carry more muscle than fat. Those pulses speed through water and trip on fat. How fast those pulses move determines your fat-to-muscle ratio. If you were to study Lance Armstrong or Michael Phelps in the lab, they'd be the poster boys for the Water Secret. So would Dara Torres, the woman who claimed an Olympic silver medal in swimming at age forty-two.

The lesson: *the more muscle you have, the better your chance of supporting cellular water. Exercise ultimately fosters hydration; the fitter you are, the less water you need to drink*. (This has nothing to do with "bulking up." When you build lean muscle, you melt away fat and uncover a toned, healthy, and *hydrated* body. No wonder people glow after exercise!) Being physically active also will spill over into other aspects of your life that honor the Water Secret. As you shape up, you'll reach for healthier foods, and generally feel motivated to pay greater attention to your lifestyle habits. There's nothing I can do to get you to move more other than to offer some tips and words of inspiration, plus reveal more alarming truths to the connections among health, hydration, and aging with regard to exercise. That's what follows in this chapter.

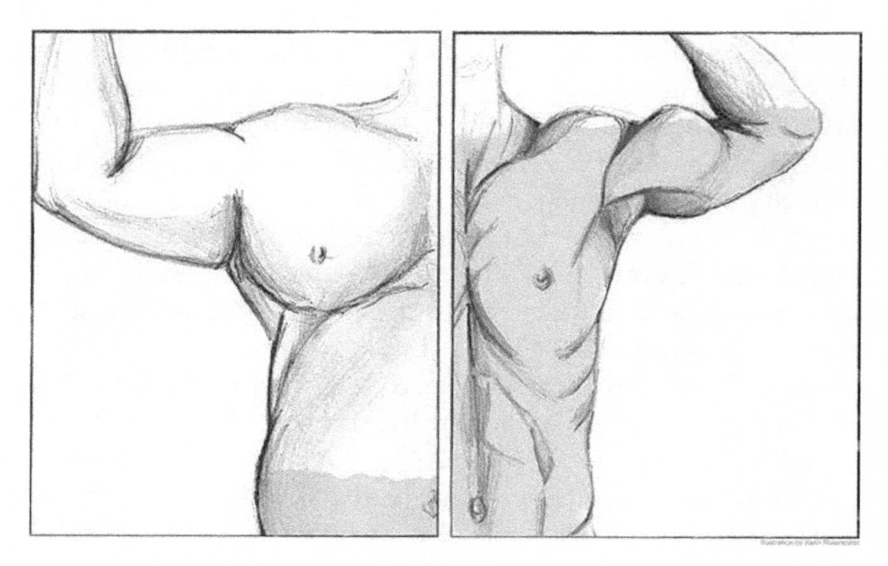

A lean, toned body will hold more water than a flabby, unfit body.

Fit Fact

If you encourage a completely sedentary person to walk around the block at a good clip, he'd be much fitter—and more positively hydrated—the next day because his cells will have responded in ways that are seemingly unimaginable. The body, as science continues to understand in the lab, is a remarkable machine.

Get Off the Dreadmill

Think about the last time you tried to "get more active" and it failed. You kept up a routine for a few weeks, maybe right after New Year's, and then suddenly it was June and you didn't want to be seen in a bathing suit. You don't remember when you fell off the wagon, but it happened. The problem for anyone trying to get active is not so much the start part as it is the *sustaining* part. At my Inclusive Health Spa, fitness and lifestyle experts help clients create a personalized, realistic plan that can be maintained. For some, that means participating in group classes at a local gym or swimming; for others, it means spending more time gardening, taking up yoga, power walking around the mall, or loading a workout DVD in the family room. There is no one-size-fits-all program, so stop beating yourself up for falling off wagons that you never should have been on. The time has come to figure out what you love to do that achieves the following: (1) gets your blood running physically and psychologically, and (2) works your muscles so that if you really pushed yourself, you'd feel a tad sore the next day.

Giving you a specific exercise protocol is beyond the scope of this book, and if you're looking for one, you're not getting the message. The goal is to align what *you* love to do with being more physical. You don't have to sweat it out on a "dreadmill" to gain health or be passionate about triathlons, like Kate. The people who boost their Phase Angles and achieve optimal levels of hydration (and health) find activities they love to do and commit to doing them more often. Simple as that.

In fact, whether you're currently active or not, get out a pen or pencil and answer the following question: if you had absolutely no obligations tomorrow, what would you do?

In my experience, the answer leads to physical activities. They may not be traditional exercises such as cycling, doing an aerobics class, or using the elliptical machine, but chances are they involve activity, maybe even the outdoors. Give yourself permission to move away from traditional formats of exercise that have never worked for you in the long run, and open yourself up to exploring opportunities to get active in other, more creative ways that really move you from the inside out. You'll keep coming back to doing them repeatedly. Remember, exercise should be about pleasure, not pain (though getting sore muscles once in a while can be a very good thing; more on that below).

Not All Fat Is Created Equal

I am reminded every day that not all fat is created equal. I also am reminded that looks can be deceiving. A seemingly lean and skinny person can score low on the Phase Angle test, as well as show higher than average body fat in the body composition analysis. I call this the Twiggy-Fat Syndrome, characterized by a low body-mass index but a high fat content. People with this syndrome typically starve their cells of much-needed nutrients, forcing their bodies into starvation mode whereby they hold tightly onto fat and cannot burn energy efficiently. On the other hand, a person who carries a little extra weight but who engages in physical exercise regularly will score much higher than a sedentary, unfit individual, who has less muscle mass. Muscle is heavier than fat pound for pound because it holds more water.

In the past decade scientists have uncovered a wealth of knowledge about types of fat on the body. Like cholesterol, there are good and bad types. Just last year researchers discovered an alarming difference between brown, or "good," fat, and the more predominant bad fat, which tends to be white or yellow and collects around the waistline. Brown fat, which actually has a brownish tint to it, is stored mostly around the neck and under the collarbone (so, to a large extent, it's invisible). This fat encourages the body to burn calories to generate body heat, and plays an important role in keeping infants warm (infants, as we all know, have fatty necks). Until very recently we believed that this fat was gone by adulthood or no longer active. Much to the contrary, it may have a huge role in our ability to stay lean as adults. These recent studies found that lean people have far more brown fat than overweight and obese people, especially among older folks. Unlike its bad-fat counterpart, brown fat burns far more calories and generates more body heat when people are in a cooler environment. Women are more likely to have it than men, and women's deposits are larger and more active.

The unhealthy fat that collects around the waistline is often referred to as *visceral* fat, because it collects around the "viscera"—your vital organs such as your heart, liver, and lungs. And it doesn't just sit there. Visceral fat is metabolically active, but instead of burning lots of calories it prefers to release chemicals that affect your metabolism—negatively. Excess calories stored as body fat generate hormones that can cause weight *gain* while preventing the production of healthy substances that can lead to weight *loss*. We are just beginning to understand how visceral fat can change the body's chemistry and work against any attempts to lose weight and fight disease.

Visceral fat is an age-maker—it wreaks havoc on our livers and has been linked to a slew of health problems, including heart disease, diabetes, some forms of cancer, and a cluster of risk factors called metabolic syndrome, which increases the chance of developing these diseases. It should come as no surprise that the more visceral fat you have, the lower the amount of cellular water you'll hold. I've witnessed this countless times in my practice and lab. Remember, muscle—not fat—is the ultimate compartment for healthy water. Fatty tissue doesn't contain very much water. This explains why women are more affected by alcohol than men are. If a man and a woman of the same weight but different body compositions were to drink the same amount of alcohol, the woman likely would feel its effects more strongly. Because women have a higher percentage of body fat, they cannot "dilute" consumed alcohol in the muscle mass the way a man with more muscle mass can. Her fat mass will not absorb very much alcohol, so the alcohol gets distributed in a smaller percentage of the total body mass (resulting in a higher blood alcohol content).

Visceral fat is not a problem just for overweight or obese people. You can be thin and still have visceral fat if you're not fit. While abdominal fat is usually visible, visceral fat can be hidden deep inside an outwardly "thin" person. The same holds true for fat that can line blood vessels, restrict blood flow, and damage the cardiovascular system.

Because visceral fat is the most dangerous kind of fat, doctors have grown more concerned about waist size than the number on the scale, which can be very deceiving. Who would you rather be: a 140-pound person with 30 percent body fat, or a 145-pound person with 20 percent body fat and

The Water Taxi

Visceral fat isn't stuck to you forever. Luckily, it responds very quickly to diet and exercise. It literally melts away when we control calories and get our bodies moving. This then paves the way to boosting cellular water. Water is the best vehicle of all for transporting fat, which makes hydration even more important. Put simply, if you want to burn fat, it must be able to be broken down and used for energy. This process, which entails a series of cellular functions, of course requires water. If the water in your blood drops below normal levels, it will pull water from your muscles to support the flow necessary in the blood. When this happens, dehydration occurs. The most fat a person can lose in a week is roughly three pounds. If you lose more than that, it's most likely water loss.

A body in motion tends to stay in motion. And when you stay in motion, you stay hydrated. Sounds counterintuitive, but it's fact, given the magic of muscle mass.

toned, shapely muscles? I think you'd pick the latter, and you'd look and feel a lot better, too. The secret to targeting that visceral fat? All you have to do is what I've already explained: move more. Eat more water, which will automatically help you cut calories and bathe your cells in the nutritious water that will speed up your metabolism and help to burn stored fat.

The Hydrating Magic of Muscle

Every year after age twenty-five, our body's composition begins to shift quite dramatically. We gain, on average, about one pound of body weight each year and lose a third to a half pound of muscle. As a result, our resting metabolism decreases approximately 0.5 percent annually. So unless you downshift your caloric intake as your metabolism slows down, you'll experience frustrating weight gain. Is this reversible? Absolutely, especially since much of this slowdown is self-perpetuated. Lifestyle changes later in life involving kids, work, and hectic schedules have more and more people doing less physically.

Women have special challenges in the fat versus muscle department. Physiological differences are to blame, as men have ten times more testosterone than women, making it so much easier for a man to build muscle. In addition, recent research suggests that women on average will lose muscle mass twice as fast as men of the same age, and that can make a huge difference in women's ability to lose or at least maintain weight. Add to that a woman's natural comparative disadvantage building muscle mass, and you can see why women have a harder time losing weight and keeping it off than men do.

In my studies with the Water Secret, a person's basal metabolic rate increases as the body becomes more efficient and positively hydrated. Your basal metabolic rate is the energy, measured in calories, that your body needs daily for your cells to function properly and to stay alive. It's what you burn without exerting any effort. Most women need a daily average of 1,500 to 1,800 calories; men need 1,600 to 2,200. Of course, this depends on activity levels, body size, and body type. To lose a pound of fat, you have to burn 3,500 more calories than you consume. For example, if you cut back on calories and increase your exercise so that you create a 500-calorie daily deficit, you'd burn enough extra fat to lose a pound in a week.

The math is straightforward, but the body seems to be anything but. People who go to extremes to lose weight quickly often impair their fat metabolism by cutting too far back on calories, which forces the body into starvation mode. When this happens, the body holds on tightly to fat and burns up muscle tissue for energy—two counterproductive events to fat loss and overall health. What's more, while it's true that in theory a calorie is a calorie, the body responds differently to the source of calories. Eating a candy bar that is loaded with refined sugar and unhealthy fat will cause a spike in insulin, which triggers storage of those calories in fat cells. Eating a turkey sandwich on whole grain with bell peppers, sprouts, and avocados, on the other hand, doesn't cause a spike and requires time and an expenditure of energy to break down its proteins, healthy fats, and complex carbohydrates. The sandwich will keep your energy balanced, support your muscles, and hydrate—rather than dehydrate—you.

People forget how valuable muscle mass is to quality of life, longevity, and the ability to maximize metabolism. Certainly genetics and special conditions such as thyroid issues can come into play when we look at weight gain and metabolic rates, but the overriding factor is muscle mass. Unlike fat, muscle is a high-maintenance tissue. It requires a lot of energy to keep it in good working order, which is why lean, more muscular people have an easier time burning calories at rest than do people with higher proportions of body fat. And it's not just about the muscle fibers that allow us to move and exercise. Think about the involuntary muscle activities that go on all the time: your heart, which itself is a muscle, pumps oxygen and nutrients to cells; muscle action pumps lymph through your lymphatic system as part of your immune system; breathing depends on muscles to deliver oxygen; and muscle activity in the skin allows us to sweat and maintain our temperature. Muscle is in constant use by the body to keep it alive and well. Muscle burns calories, whereas fat just stores them. This is why the more lean muscle you have, the faster your metabolism will be. It's the main determinant of whether your metabolism is humming at a hundred miles an hour or crawling at a tenth that rate.

> In most people, muscle strength peaks at about ages twenty to thirty, then gradually decreases. Without strength training, most people experience a 30 percent loss in overall strength by age seventy.

Although losing a fraction of muscle mass each year may seem minuscule, it adds up to be quite significant—translating to about a 1 to 2 percent loss of strength each year. With this loss of muscle strength, we tend to spontaneously become less active because daily activities become more difficult and exhausting to perform.

The Bone-us of Strength Training

Strength training gets so much attention in fitness circles because it supports lean muscle mass and can help to increase muscle mass, strength, and bone health. While aerobic exercise improves cardiovascular fitness and burns calories (and is essential to any fitness program), it has minimal influence on muscle mass, strength, and bone health. Strength training can provide up to a 15 percent increase in metabolic rate, which is enormously helpful for weight loss and long-term weight control. While aerobic exercise burns fat chiefly *during* exercise, strength training utilizes fat hours *after* exercise. The burn keeps going for longer than you're working out. Strength training also has been shown to increase bone mass, which is extremely important for women because of the increased risk of developing the brittle-bone disease osteoporosis. The muscles you engage when you lift a weight puts pressure on your bones, forcing them to get stronger. In fact, recent studies have shown that loss of bone density may be a better predictor of death from atherosclerosis (hardening of the arteries) than cholesterol levels. And there are additional benefits. Strength training is an effective antidepressant and can even improve sleep quality.

The more muscle you have, the more calories you burn throughout the day—whether you are walking, vacuuming, or sleeping. This is because muscle is metabolically active. Stored fat, on the other hand, is less metabolically active, uses very little energy, and therefore burns minimal calories. Muscle equals hydration. Fat equals dehydration.

Strength training can be done with free weights (barbells and dumbbells) or with universal gyms that work various parts of

Curl Up in the Morning

A great way to start three of your days per week is to roll right into a bicep curl routine. Keep a pair of weights under your bed (start with three to five pounds) and pull them out after you stretch your arms as you get out of bed. Complete two sets of fifteen repetitions (with your hands at your sides, each hand holding a weight, curl them up slowly toward your chest, then down slowly). You'll soon begin to see more definition and feel stronger in your upper arms.

your body in a more controlled way. It should be done two or three times a week for about thirty minutes each time. Don't use weights every day. An every-other-day schedule allows your muscles to recover; try not to exercise the same muscles two days in a row.

Get Sore to Get Stronger

As you age, your body's ability to produce an adequate supply of joint fluids, such as hyaluronic acid, diminishes, which leads to "unlubed" joints that can cause pain, inflammation, and arthritis. This prevents a person from exercising, which further weakens joints, and the condition deteriorates. The key is to stay mobile and keep your joints moving. Like the old saying goes, if you don't use it, you lose it.

It also pays to be sore once in a while after a tough workout. All improvement in any muscle function comes from stressing and recovering. Let's say that you exercise hard enough to make your muscles burn during the exercise. The burning is a sign that you are stressing your muscles. The next day, your muscles feel sore because they have been worked and need time to recover. Scientists call this DOMS, or delayed onset muscle soreness.

It takes at least eight hours to feel this type of soreness. You finish a workout and feel great; then you get up the next morning and your exercised muscles feel heavy and achy. We used to think that next-day muscle soreness was caused by a buildup of lactic acid in muscles, but now we know that lactic acid has nothing to do with it. Next-day muscle soreness is caused by damage to the muscle fibers themselves, due in large part to inflammation as a result of microscopic tears of the muscle fibers. Muscle biopsies taken on the day after hard exercise show bleeding and disruption of the z-band filaments that hold muscle fibers together as they slide over each other during a contraction. Is this a bad thing? Far from it.

This muscle pain is a normal response to unusual exertion and is part of an adaptation process that leads to greater stamina and strength as the muscles recover and build bigger cells that can hold more nutrients and water. It's not the same as the muscle pain or fatigue you experience during exercise. This delayed pain is also very different from the acute, sudden pain of an injury such as a muscle strain or sprain, which is marked by an abrupt, specific, and sudden pain during activity and often causes swelling or bruising.

How do you know how far to take your workouts? Remember that you don't have to be training for an Olympic event to gain fitness. Next-day muscle soreness can be used as a guide to getting into and, more importantly, staying in shape. All you have to do is go out one day and exercise right up to the burn, back off when your muscles really start to burn, then pick up the pace again and exercise to the burn. This can entail simply power walking on hills. Do this exercise-to-the-burn and recover until your muscles start to feel stiff, then stop the workout. Depending on how sore your muscles feel, take the next day off or go at a very slow pace. Do not attempt to get that burning sensation back during exercise until the soreness has gone away completely. Most athletes take a very hard workout one day, go easy for one to seven days afterward, and then take a hard workout again. World-class marathon runners run very fast only twice a week. The best weight lifters lift very heavy only

Strength in Numbers: The More You Move, the More You Burn

- General dancing: 975 calories per hour
- Power walking: 600 calories per hour
- Heavy or major cleaning of the house (for example, washing the car, washing windows, cleaning the garage) with vigorous effort: 450 calories per hour
- Clearing dishes from the table, washing dishes, and walking: 375 calories per hour
- Watching a movie: 150 calories per hour

Numbers based on a 150-pound person.

The other numbers you need to know: according to updated guidelines issued by the American College of Sports Medicine, engaging in moderate-intensity physical activity for 150 minutes per week (30 minutes per day, 5 days a week) may offer a great start to getting fit, but it won't cut the mustard in terms of long-term weight loss and management. Greater amounts of weekly physical activity—on the order of 250 minutes or more per week—is more realistic. This means 50 minutes a day, 5 days a week. Remember, though, that it doesn't have to happen all at once.

once every two weeks. High jumpers jump for height only once a week. Shot-putters throw for distance only once a week. Don't forget: exercise training is done by stressing and recovering.

Sitting Pretty: The Unlikely Source of Power in Posture

Here's an idea few people think about every day: paying attention to posture, especially when you're sitting at a desk hammering away at work. Posture, which is essentially how you hold yourself up and position your body, helps your muscles to *stay* strong and helps your digestive system to work at peak performance. A healthy spine supports your weight and protects your nerves and organs, enabling you to move easily throughout your day. It also protects the spinal cord and nerves that relay messages between your brain and your body.

Yoga and Pilates can help you focus on posture and improve upon it, or you can simply imagine someone pulling a string up through your body from your feet to your head. See if you can go a day without slouching forward or leaning back.

Chart Progress, but Don't Aim for Perfection

One of my favorite sayings is "Don't be perfect; live longer." The great thing about exercise is that its benefits accumulate. You don't have to go full-out every day of the week for an obscene number of hours. Just twenty minutes here, a stair-climb there, and ten minutes lifting weights in front of the television a few times a week can have immediate impacts. The more fit you become, the easier your exercises will feel and the more you'll want to further challenge your body. Remember, too, that as your fitness level increases, your capacity to stay hydrated also will increase naturally as you gain water-holding, fat-burning muscle mass. You may find that you don't need to drink so much during or after your workouts.

I have discovered that patients who chart their activities each week in a journal are the most successful with maintaining a personal program and knowing when to up the ante. For example, if you don't feel 100 percent on a Tuesday, and you look at your journal and see that you haven't moved your body in any significant way since last Wednesday, you know that you need to schedule more activity in the coming days. It also may help to keep track of your food intake for the same reason: you'll be able to spot days when your meals aren't ideal. No one is perfect every day, but as you chart your habits you'll recognize progress at the same time and realize an enormous sense of satisfaction that can be very rewarding and motivating.

Boost Your Mood with Movement, Not Food

The average American is exposed to about 3,900 calories a day through TV, radio, and print ads. Brain researchers increasingly report that fat-and-sugar combinations in particular light up the brain's dopamine pathway, which is a pleasure-sensing spot implicated in people's addictions to alcohol or drugs. The more we see food, the more we want to eat it. A recent survey found that 36 percent of people felt an urge to eat after watching others do so on TV. Just thinking about a food increases the likelihood that you'll eat it. The good news: that's also true of healthy foods. So looking at a delicious salad or thinking how you'll feel after you eat it may be enough to take your mind off some restaurant chain advertising a bottomless bowl of fettuccine Alfredo. More good news: physical activity targets the dopamine pathway, too, and can be a healthy distraction when junk food is in plain view.

And sometimes *slowing down* is the secret to getting fitter. If you find yourself juggling too many to-dos and losing out on quality time for yourself, you can easily watch days or even weeks go by where your good intentions fall by the wayside. Set some boundaries and tell yourself that for every week you don't get enough physical activity, you'll take a two- or even three-hour time-out from your normal routine to tend to your body's needs. Use that time-out to engage in a physical activity of your choice, and combine that with another activity you find stress-relieving and pleasurable. Maybe it's shopping with a friend, cooking, or reading a book.

No Time, No Energy, No Way

If you can't fathom doing any physical exercise most days of the week between your work and family life, you're among the millions of people who struggle to schedule regular physical activity into their busy lives. Not having time and not feeling up to it are the two biggest complaints I hear.

The secret is to find what you love to do and make that a priority in your list of tasks for the week. Don't force yourself to engage in any activities that bore you or mentally drain you. Gyms and group exercise classes are not for everyone. Also bear in mind that exercise is invigorating. As soon as you get your circulation going, those feelings of "I'm too tired" usually fade away as endorphins begin to take over. Try moving your workouts to the morning, when the day's events haven't kicked in to disrupt you or wear you down. The first five minutes are the hardest, but once you get over that initial hump, the body takes over. And if you do find yourself chronically tired, then I'd stop to ask why. Chronic exhaustion isn't a sign of health. You would do well to examine your lifestyle, priorities, and attempts to reduce your stress load.

Hope for Athletes, Soldiers, and Even You

Aside from the message about moving more in your life to support hydration naturally, here's a final thought to consider. When your body is equipped with the right tools it needs to operate, which entail nutrients and strong muscle tissue, among other things, it won't have to bother you to seek hydration through copious water drinking. As we saw with Kate at the beginning of this chapter, not having to carry or stop for water made a difference in her performance. Recently I wrote a paper about the potential benefits of the Water Secret on soldiers, who often endure tough terrain and can face dehydration. It's common knowledge that success or failure hinges on the strength, endurance, and mental acuity of the individual carrying out a mission. But it's not commonly thought that soldiers, like athletes, can enhance their hydration capacity by focusing on efficient sources of key cell-fortifying nutrients rather than just carrying cumbersome and heavy jugs of water.

Since the beginning of time, the human body has been used as a tool for survival and achievement. Through disciplined exercise, athletes mold muscles and train their reflexes to reach goals and outdo previous records. In the military, rigorous training and physical drills sharpen soldiers who, in times of war, must become formidable athletes as they face situations requiring unwavering perseverance. Countless studies have explored methods to maintain and increase peak performance, stamina, and strength; prevent injury; and sharpen mind-body coordination in an effort to build better athletes. These studies in athletic training easily translate to military personnel and can provide officers with the necessary tools to fortify their regiments. At the core of these methods, clinical experiments have indicated that the answer to achieving and surmounting athletic goals lies at the cellular level. At this level, nutrients assist in making cell membranes more resistant to water loss, adding to a soldier's or athlete's overall stability from basic tissue components to major systems and even emotions—all of which are of great importance to athletes and soldiers.

And this should be of great importance to you, too, even though you may not call yourself and athlete or a soldier. If an inclusive approach can provide athletes with an edge in training and soldiers a strategic advantage, then imagine what it can do for you.

CHAPTER 7

Why Skin Care Is Health Care

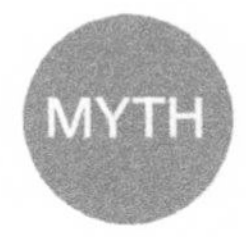

Your looks are mostly genetically determined.

It's not unusual for my patients to hear the following from friends once they've followed the Water Secret for just a few weeks: "You look so good . . . so . . . *healthy*. What are you doing?"

I often remind people that "skin care is health care." I can't emphasize this enough: Your skin is connected to every part of your body, and as your body's largest organ, it's a mirror of your inner health. In other words, *how hydrated your internal cells are can be seen on the outside because your skin offers a window into cell conditions deep within your body*. So what's going on inside can be seen on the outside, and vice versa. Again, this reiterates the connectedness of the whole body, from the color of your cheeks to the pulse of your blood in your intestines.

Think about the last time you were sick with a cold or flu bug. You *looked* ill even though the actual infection was taking place deep within your body. You probably looked pale, sallow, and dried out. But you don't necessarily have to be sick to show signs of simply not taking proper care of yourself. In this regard, beauty is not about vanity at all; beauty is an indicator of health. Beauty *is* health. Although it may appear to be merely skin deep, the skin holds an advanced degree in communications, silently telegraphing illness or health, pleasure or pain, embarrassment or enthusiasm. And if you think you've got no chance of being "beautiful" by society's standards, listen up: most of the elements of physical beauty are under your control, no matter what genetic hand your parents dealt you.

Because of the duality of internal health and skin health, when you make your skin healthy, you make every other organ in your body healthy, too. And just as the goal of the Cellular Water Secret Diet on internal cells is to improve cellular hydration, the skin health goal of the diet is to boost its barrier function and help the skin's cells hold as much water as possible.

The cosmetic and beauty industry is enormous, and walking into a department store's or retail chain's overflowing beauty section can be intimidating and overwhelming. Too much to choose from. Too many claims, promises, and hype. Which products are the best? Which are worth the price? Does it matter based on your skin type, age, and lifestyle? These are among the questions I'm going to address in this chapter, giving you an easy guide for taking care of your skin in the most practical way possible.

> You have no control over the cards that are dealt to you. But, you do have control over how you play your hand.

About Skin

Skin does more than present your face to the world. It plays a vital role in the maintenance of physical and mental health. Not only does it act as an insulator, shock absorber, and wound healer, it's also your greatest and most loyal protector. When people hear the word *immunity*, their initial thoughts often gravitate toward vaccines, white blood cells, and infectious diseases. However, the body's first and most influential line of immunity defense is the skin, which is why improving the integrity of the skin's immunity affords the body better armor against invading bacteria, viruses, and toxins that can trigger disease, while also reducing the visible signs of aging.

About 70 percent of skin is water. Because of its sponge-like abilities, which allow it to absorb water and hydrating elements from the outside world, it can also absorb enough energy from UV rays to make vitamin D, or absorb too much UV energy and cause serious damage. The skin is also in tune with what's going on inside your body. Skin participates in fighting off infections; warming you up; cooling you down; and, of course, keeping you hydrated. Skin is not an idle blanket. It's an incredibly dynamic organ, and it continually regenerates itself so it has a completely new population of cells every four to five weeks.

> Your skin is your largest organ, taking up about 16 percent of your total body weight. It contains hair, oil and sweat glands, nerves, and blood vessels.

And, as you'll learn in the next chapter, the skin and the body are connected through an elaborate relationship called the neuro-immuno-cutaneous-endocrine network, which makes it such a marvelous communicator. Dermatologists have long recognized neuropsychological connections between the appearance of the skin, perception of beauty, and health. But it doesn't take a medical degree to understand this connection just from casual observation alone. Anyone who has experienced skin problems such as acne or eczema during acutely stressful time periods can attest to this fact. What you can't necessarily see, though, is the cellular water loss in the skin that can exacerbate flare-ups and generally bring down an otherwise youthful appearance.

> Beautiful skin is healthy skin. Healthy skin is beautiful.

About Face

Your skin might look like a single piece of wrapping paper keeping the internal goods inside, but skin is one of the body's most complex and multitasking organs. It holds an array of compounds that enable it to do its job, including proteins; amino acids; vitamins; trace minerals; antioxidants; fats; sugars; and, of course, water. Like a hard-working machine that's turned on 24/7, it needs more and more input and maintenance as you age because it gets worn down through use and becomes more inefficient and less reliable. The skin you see is just the top layer, but skin is made of many layers that go much deeper, the lowest of which anchors itself to a still lower, fatty layer.

Skin care products and treatments have evolved considerably in direct proportion to scientific research. After decades in the industry, I've seen a lot of products hit the shelves, some of which are inexpensive and can work wonders on the skin, while others fall short of their promises and can cost a small fortune. As a dedicated researcher and formulator, I've prided myself on bringing the best, most transformative products to people with attention to details—including price, effectiveness, and safety. Fad and trends will always come and go, but real solutions based on real science will always be treasured and find a lasting place in the market.

Today's dermatologists and plastic surgeons offer an enormous number of treatments that can help improve the appearance of aging skin. Understanding the limitations of these procedures can help you have realistic expectations. A face-lift, for instance, will tighten skin and reposition the underlying tissue; resurfacing techniques to remove the top layer of skin can erase fine lines and hyperpigmentation areas but won't alter deep wrinkles. Botox temporarily paralyzes muscles, so you are unable to contract them, thus giving the illusion of smoother skin. Wrinkle fillers such as collagen, fat, and hyaluronic acid gel temporarily plump the depression of a fine line or scar or a hollow area, again giving the impression of smoothness or fullness. All of these measures help you appear more youthful. If you do choose any of these procedures with the help of a dermatologist, the strategies in this book will enhance their results. But keep in mind that they are all temporary fixes; they will not stop the march of time and the natural aging process. The practices aligned with the Water Secret, on the other hand, will equip your body with the tools it needs to improve, heal, and defend your skin against the ravages of time and age. Whereas many cosmetic medical treatments today cover up or mask signs of age and skin damage, the Water Secret helps to attack the aging process at the cellular level. You would do well to incorporate its strategies into your life not only to improve your skin's appearance but also to improve your skin's inherent health and function. No procedure or treatment can do that.

Just as the Water Secret encourages you to strengthen and heal your internal cells and connective tissue to maintain water levels and functionality, the Water Secret will guide you to seek out topical ingredients to do the same from the outside, strengthening and healing your skin to prevent water loss. This will help you to be less susceptible to environmental damage and premature aging and give you firmer, healthier, and more radiant skin.

Of all the skin care ingredients touted to make you look prettier, the ones that have the most profound impact on skin health are based in real science and include the hydroxy acids, topical antioxidants (including vitamin C), and peptides.

Skin through the Ages

Troublesome teens: Skin is taut and wrinkle-free during this age, but acne is a common experience for many. Breakouts are usually associated with hormonal fluctuations as the body goes through puberty. When puberty is over, though, the acne lessens or even disappears for most people.

(*continued*)

Roaring twenties: This decade starts out with a bang of good, young-looking skin but soon starts to show signs of adulthood as skin starts to lose collagen and elastin. The beginnings of wrinkles are visible, particularly in the eye region (known as "crow's-feet"). Most twentysomethings have uniform skin pigmentation, but if contraceptive pills are used or a woman becomes pregnant, some discoloration may occur. The decline in hormone levels begins for many women in their twenties, and imbalances during a woman's cycle can trigger skin symptoms at both ends of the spectrum such as acne and oiliness, or dryness and dull skin. Declining hormone levels also cause the skin to thin, which accelerates with age. We lose 1 percent of collagen every year starting at age twenty.

Thirties-plus: The natural decline in the skin's elasticity continues alongside a decline in natural hormones. There is more skin thinning, dead skin cell buildup, and skin discoloration. Sometimes acne is present, but pimples are cystlike, long-lasting, and deep. While the onset of menopause usually occurs between the ages of forty-five and fifty-five, some women in their early thirties experience menopausal sleeplessness, weight gain, irritability, temporary memory loss, hot flashes, brittle hair, and dry skin. Irregular periods, excessive hair growth in unexpected places such as the chin, and acne could indicate polycystic ovarian syndrome. Women who are nutritionally deficient, smoke, or who never have had children will approach menopause at an earlier age than they normally would have without these factors. Constant, unrelenting stress has also been shown to accelerate hormonal aging, as stress hormone overproduction can cause symptoms associated with adrenal gland fatigue. Adrenal fatigue has been described in the medical literature to be a factor in many related conditions, including fibromyalgia, hypothyroidism, chronic fatigue syndrome, arthritis, and premature menopause, and may cause many undesirable side effects such as acne, hair loss, depression, weight gain, a decline in the immune system, and insomnia.

Nature's Acids Are Nature's Antidotes to Aging: Who Knew an Acid Could Feel So Good?

Alpha-hydroxy acids, sometimes known as fruit acids because they are found naturally in fruit, were truly the first *cosmeceutical* ingredients—ingredients that are more active than cosmetics, but not so active that they have uncomfortable or harmful side effects, as drugs do. In 1989 I was among the first to bring alpha-hydroxy acids to the field of dermatology and topical skin care. The most popular alpha-hydroxy acids for the skin include glycolic acid, from sugarcane, and lactic acid, from milk. Beta-hydroxy acids, notably salicylic acid, eventually entered the arena as well, and because BHAs are oil-soluble, they can help to clean out clogged pores. With hydroxy acids, "feel good" facials became true treatments because they speed up skin shedding, removing the dead, dry cells from the surface of the skin and spurring new cell turnover. Hydroxy acids will prepare your skin to accept moisturizing ingredients and nutrients, leaving it smooth and hydrated. They also can help dry skin to hold on to moisture. Anything you rub into your newly exfoliated skin will penetrate more deeply and be more effective.

Add to cart: An AHA/BHA exfoliating cleanser is a great product to have and use twice weekly on your face and any other body parts you choose. Hydroxy acids are now ubiquitous in facial creams and cleansers, and can reduce the appearance of fine lines and wrinkles. If your skin is sensitive, you may want to start with a beta-hydroxy acid formula first and then try one with the AHA-BHA combination. Alpha-hydroxy acids can be irritating for some; you don't want to remove dead cells faster than your body can produce new ones. Some initial irritation or redness is to be expected, so try a smaller amount or use just once a week to start. If your skin never seems to get used to it, opt for exfoliants that use gentle grains such as sugar; salt; oatmeal; ground jojoba seeds; or small, synthetic beads. The best way to apply an exfoliant on your face is with your hands. Loofahs and exfoliating mitts are best left for your larger body parts with more abrasion-tolerant skin.

You also may choose to visit a dermatologist or an aesthetician who can perform a more rigorous treatment using a glycolic peel, which penetrates the skin deeply with a higher concentration of acids, or microdermabrasion. A microdermabrasion treatment involves a machine that basically removes the outermost layer of skin. These procedures, however, are likely to cause a brief period of redness and irritation, so don't schedule them the day of a big event. Give your skin a week to recover and really glow.

Exfoliants are not limited to use on the face. You can exfoliate any body parts you choose. You'll find exfoliants labeled for facial and/or body use.

Dry Skin Brushing

Another way to exfoliate your entire body is to save the wash for your face but try dry skin brushing on other body parts before stepping into the shower or bath. Not only does regular use of this technique remove old dead and dying cells around your body, it also increases the blood flow and stimulates the lymphatic system's ability to remove built-up toxins. That's right: this is a way to enhance your body's natural detoxification system while exfoliating every square inch for a healthy glow. Get a brush designed just for this at your local beauty store or pharmacy. They typically will have a long handle to reach various parts and have natural bristles made from goat, boar, or vegetables. Sweep the brush once or twice over your body, always working toward your heart. So if you're brushing your legs, work your way up. Use gentle, circular motions on your belly.

Homemade Scrub and Detox Bath

Try mixing your own natural body scrub in the kitchen by combining Turbinado sugar, safflower oil, and coarsely ground coffee, which will help soften and cleanse pores. Draw a warm bath with Epsom salts. This will help you to revive muscles and depuff skin. Then, when you get out, lather more safflower oil onto the roughest, driest parts of your skin below the neckline. Safflower oil is rich in moisturizing linoleic acid. Or you can try extra-virgin organic coconut oil, sold at health food stores. These will melt into your skin.

Topical Antioxidants

The discovery of hydroxy acids stimulated more thinking on how to protect, nourish, and condition newly exfoliated skin to exponentially increase and maintain results. Dermatologists began touting the virtues of sunscreen to protect newly exfoliated skin. The skin care industry followed their lead and added sunscreen as a necessary step in skin treatments. More than just offering SPF protection, however, cosmetic chemists started down another important path of study. The new, uncharted track was the study of topical vitamins such as A, C, and E. These three antioxidants became the nourishing triad of ingredients du jour. Many moisturizers featured these vitamins and sunscreen ingredients. Whole lines were produced featuring antioxidants as the star ingredients.

Antioxidants have been a hot topic in the health world for several years, and my work with them dates back to the early 1990s. Loosely, an antioxidant is a substance that helps create a barrier from free-radical damage, also known as the decaying process of oxidation. Oxidation is what causes most of the visible signs of aging in the skin, even though oxidation itself is going on at a very small, atomic level that you really can't see. It's what happens when molecules in the body lose an electron and become unstable. Those renegade electrons act like loose cannons, which then seek out other molecules, crashing into them, stealing more electrons, and spreading more damage. A great majority of the free-radical sources comes from your environment—things such as UV radiation from the sun, pollution, and cigarette smoke.

It's impossible to avoid the creation of all free-radical damage, since day-to-day bodily functions such as digestion and breathing produce free radicals. They are facts of life, but they should be controlled, to the extent possible, to reduce their ability to inflict damage on your cells. The only molecules that can lose electrons without becoming unstable are antioxidant molecules. They have the unique ability to stop oxidation in its tracks by disarming free radicals. Like a waiter serving food to hungry, edgy people, antioxidants travel with extra electrons to pass out and restabilize molecules. Different types of antioxidants work in their own way, given their special strengths. Ginkgo biloba, for example, seems to provide most of its benefits to the brain, while coenzyme Q10 is most effective in the heart. Green tea contains catechins, antioxidants that have been shown to reduce inflammation and inhibit cancer formations on skin. In the laboratory, tea catechins inhibit cancer growth by scavenging oxidants before cell injuries occur, reducing the incidence and size of chemically induced tumors, and inhibiting the growth of tumor cells. In studies of liver, skin, and stomach cancer, chemically induced tumors were shown to decrease in size in mice that were fed green and black tea. Antioxidants come in a variety of forms, including vitamins and minerals. Your body can create some antioxidants, but others must be obtained from food and supplements. Cutting-edge scientific breakthroughs have allowed us to infuse these free-radical fighters directly into the skin with topical creams rich in antioxidants that work best in the skin and can penetrate deeply.

> Antioxidants, in general, have been found to stimulate collagen production, so they are key ingredients in antiaging protocols.

The Top Ten

Look for moisturizers containing ingredients on the following list, since all of them can fight oxidative stress that ages us internally and externally:

1. Pomegranate extract
2. Goji berry extract
3. Vitamin C
4. Vitamin E
5. Aloe vera
6. Zinc
7. Licorice extract
8. Green tea
9. Durian
10. Grape seed extract

The best hydrating ingredients include sodium PCA, hyaluronic acid, glycerine, and goji berry extract.

More powerful antioxidants are discovered every day, and most recently we've seen pomegranate, goji berry, ellagic acid, and green tea extract incorporated into topical formulas. Cosmetics chemists continue to study ingredient percentages and optimal vehicles for antiaging antioxidants. In the midst of all of this antioxidant study, one topical vitamin has clearly stood out: vitamin C, a multitasker in the skin. In your outermost skin layer, where there is five times more vitamin C than in the deeper skin layers, it performs several functions. It helps prevent water loss and therefore maintains the skin's barrier function. It's involved in collagen- and elastin-building. And it deactivates unstable free radicals before they can cause too much damage. There also is increasing evidence that vitamin C shields the skin from the sun's burning rays, especially when it's applied in high concentrations or combined with vitamin E, sunscreens, and skin soothers.

Because there's a limit to how much vitamin C the body can absorb through food, researchers have discovered that if they could bypass the body and go directly to the skin, they could increase its vitamin C content more than twenty times! At first it was a guessing game with regard to percentage and type of vitamin C used. On the downside, vitamin C is a very delicate ingredient that is sensitive to light, pH, and oxidation, and it can be very unstable. It also can cause considerable irritation on skin. But through extensive research over the years, cosmetics chemists have found the answers necessary to make highly concentrated, stable products. They even figured out ways to quell skin irritation and inflammation with compatible, soothing ingredients. And all this research paved the way for top-quality products so people could safely and reliably reap the benefits of vitamin C.

Add to cart: Seek out moisturizers that contain antioxidants such as stable forms of vitamin C and others that can protect skin from sun damage, inflammation, DNA damage, and skin cancers. The list of free-radical fighters added to topicals continues to grow and includes certain ingredients in pomegranates, grape-seed extract, goji berries, green tea, dark chocolate, and coffeeberry. I recommend using a moisturizer with sunscreen—at least SPF 15—during the day, and switch to a sunscreen-free formula at night. You also may want to opt for a thicker, richer lotion at night, since your body will be in sleep mode and bringing out the troops to repair cells. Night creams contain a greater concentration of hydrating ingredients that most people don't find comfortable to wear during the day or under makeup, but they needn't be greasy or heavy. Water loss through the skin is greatest at night, which is why using a thicker formula can help prevent that kind of dehydration. The body's cells are replenished with nutrients and are being regenerated at night, so this is the time to optimize the delivery of the raw materials that skin needs. Because free-radical production is at its lowest at night, saturating the

UVA vs. UVB

Ultraviolet radiation comes in two forms: A and B. The A rays are associated with aging because their damage to the skin is what causes premature wrinkles and pigment changes. The B rays, for burning, cause the classic sunburn—inflammation and dilated blood vessels. Look for a broad-spectrum sunscreen that blocks out both UVA and UVB rays.

skin with a rich formula will also prepare you for the next day. In addition, you may choose to use a night cream that includes agents that optimize skin's sleep cycle, such as melatonin and GABA, an amino acid that has a calming effect on cells and encourages muscle relaxation to maximize the body's ability to repair and regenerate during the night.

Watering the Skin with Moisturizers

It's well known that the purpose of moisturizers is to do exactly that—bring moisture to the skin to replenish its natural moisture in the upper layers and reinforce the skin's barrier function. Picture the difference between the skin on a newborn baby and an adult. The baby's skin is supple, soft, pliable, pristine, dewy, and visibly hydrated, whereas the adult's shows signs of wear and tear. It's drier in some places and nowhere near as taut and impermeable-looking as the baby's fresh coat. When we are young, our skin is firm and intact, and its outermost layer is sturdy like a new roof. As we age, our skin's barrier function diminishes. Not only does it become filled with more dead, ineffectual cells than young, strong ones, but also the fatty layer that forms the seal between the cells becomes depleted. This leaves us vulnerable for transepidermal water loss—water essentially escapes from the skin tissue and evaporates into the air, much like heat escaping through holes in an old, beat-up roof.

This is why applying moisturizer is so important. It performs two chief tasks. First, it infuses skin with water; and second, it seals the holes between cells so you keep that water in and reduce water loss to the environment. It's important to note that no moisturizer can change the fabric of your skin; it can't affect how the skin functions at the cellular level, changing the production of collagen and repairing tissue damage per se, but a good moisturizer gives your skin the ingredients it needs to then perform its functions optimally. I recommend finding a moisturizer that contains the ultimate trio of hydrators, antioxidants, and anti-inflammatories.

Virtually all moisturizers have similar ingredients as hydrators. Humectants such as hyaluronic acid, sorbitol, glycerin, propylene glycerol, urea, and sodium lactate draw water to the skin's surface, thus increasing its water content; emollients such as lanolin, jojoba oil, isopropyl palmitate, propylene glycol linoleate, squalene, and glycerol stearates act as the lubricants on the surface to fill in the cracks between cells ready to shed; and ceramides are lipids naturally found in the skin's top layer, alongside other fats such as cholesterol and fatty acids. Ceramides are what keep moisture in the skin, and they have been used to treat eczema. And as I've mentioned, many moisturizers come with additional ingredients targeted to treat, repair, and prevent future damage. These include antioxidants, anti-inflammatories, sunscreen, and natural ingredients known to help keep skin firm and blemish-free. These natural ingredients, which can be anything from vitamin C to extracts from plants and fruits, can enhance the product's effectiveness.

> Everyone—regardless of skin type—needs to moisturize. Even people with oily, acne-prone skin need to hydrate and restore the barrier function of their skin.

Apply moisturizer every day to any area of your body that needs it. It's ideal to rub moisturizer into your skin just after washing it and patting it nearly dry so you trap some of that water.

Special Ingredients for Special Skin

Depending on your unique skin needs, you will want to consider additional ingredients and/or products that target certain skin issues. The following are some ideas:

For acne-prone skin: Unfortunately, acne is no longer just a fact of adolescent life. I see more and more of it in adults long past their teenage years (and they have wrinkles, for a double whammy). The prevalence of acne underscores the fact that acne rarely has a single cause and reiterates the whole-body connectedness. Whether a result of hormones, stress, exposure to more pollution, prescription medications such as steroids or birth control pills, genetics, or a combination thereof, acne shows up on skin, but owes its origins to somewhere else in the body. Kits that contain acne-treatment products are very effective today. They usually have a cocktail of ingredients that work on different aspects of the condition. For instance, powerful exfoliating agents help eliminate the dead skin cells that accumulate in pores or follicles. Antiseptic ingredients help remove acne-fueling bacteria. A matifying agent helps remove the excess oil on which the bacteria thrive and promote acne. And soothing agents help quell the inflammation and irritation. If you don't respond to these standard treatments, see a dermatologist who can help tailor a treatment specifically for you and consider prescription options.

For advanced aging and wrinkles: More than sixty years ago, scientists began developing synthetic forms of vitamin A called retinoids. Many have been used as drugs, and two of them—tretinoin (example brands: Retin-A, Avita, Renova) and tazarotene (example brands: Tazorac, Avage)—have proved effective not just for wrinkles but for acne, too. Prescription retinoids can smooth wrinkles, unclog pores, lighten superficial brown spots, and improve the texture of the skin. They also win the war on acne, and can be used to treat other skin conditions, such as psoriasis. Retinoids can regenerate collagen and may help prevent basal cell and squamous cell carcinomas as well. So why isn't everyone using them? For starters, these vitamin A derivatives are drugs that come with potential side effects. Some people cannot tolerate the irritation these treatments cause their face for several weeks at the start (it typically gets better as the skin adjusts). And you must keep using the product to see the results. I will prescribe these wrinkle- and acne-fighters on occasion, but I'm quick to remind my patients that they are not magic bullets. They still need to infuse their skin with antioxidants, anti-inflammatories, and hydrators. The skin becomes very sensitive to sunlight, so if you use a retinoid, you'd rub it on at night and wear a broad-spectrum sunscreen during the day, even when it's raining.

That said, less potent versions of retinoids are available now and are in many over-the-counter skin creams. I have incorporated them in many of my products. Retinols, including retinyl palmitate, are much less likely to cause irritation and have shown, over time, to be as effective as their prescription-strength counterparts. In a study presented in the journal *Archives of Dermatology*, it was reported that over-the-counter retinol use in elderly patients increased collagen production, and this resulted in making skin more resilient to injury and ulcer formation.

For hyperpigmentation: Too much pigment in your skin is what you see when you look at brown spots, splotches, and darker areas. They're all a result of too much melanin rising to your skin's surface, which also can occur as a result of pregnancy, birth control pills, sunlight, acne, and scars. Discoloration can arise at any age, but it's most likely going to show up in people past age twenty in many races, including African American, Asian, Hispanic, and Caucasian. The most effective treatment is hydroquinone, which is available in both 2 percent over the counter and 4 percent in prescription strength. It's not exactly bleach, but it lightens the skin by inhibiting the chemical reactions that create melanin, so people sometimes refer to hydroquinone as a skin-bleaching cream. Use this in the morning, ideally with a product infused with vitamin C. It can be combined with a hydroxy acid to increase cell turnover. The skin cells with the extra pigment are shed more quickly, and the pigmentation of the new skin cells is more uniform. Pregnant or nursing women should not use hydroquinone because studies have not been done to determine safety for those conditions. Hydroquinone is not too foreign to us. Most of us consume it daily in foods such as berries, coffee, wheat, and tea. If you try a hydroquinone product and don't see positive results within three months, speak with a dermatologist.

For menopausal skin: Women experiencing advanced hormonal aging at the onset of menopause have a unique set of challenges. During the years leading up to menopause, the body produces decreasing quantities of estrogen. With estrogen loss, the skin (and the body) are affected in many ways—again, reiterating the whole-body connectedness. Since the face has a high concentration of estrogen receptors, menopause may be at its most visible there. As skin becomes progressively sensitive and dry, it becomes increasingly more important to include ingredients that can hydrate, strengthen, and protect without causing irritation. Like all skin, menopausal skin needs to be infused with antioxidants, anti-inflammatories, and hydrators, but it needs products that are compatible with dry, sensitive skin and that do the job gently. Apricot, evening primrose, and borage seed oils can be incorporated to strengthen the skin's barrier function and help it stay hydrated. Superdry skin conditions will benefit from shea butter.

Gentle topical exfoliators such as papaya enzyme will help control skin discoloration, remove dead cells and excess oils that combine to create acne, and help prepare skin for firming and toning ingredients such as clove flower and iris extracts. Hair, skin, and nails—everything gets weaker with estrogen loss, so adding the cell-growth stimulant biotin as a dietary supplement is essential to restore strength.

For skin around the eyes: There's a reason why products are specifically formulated for use in the eye area. The skin around the eyes is thin and absorbs ingredients more rapidly than skin on other areas of the face. There are no oil glands in the eye area, so there is less natural lubrication. Eye creams are formulated with all these differences in mind, and often include ingredients not normally found in regular moisturizers. For example, I think a good eye cream should contain caffeine to reduce the amount of water in the spaces between the cells that cause puffiness, various peptides to support new collagen formation, vitamin C to prevent damage from free radicals, skin soothers to reduce inflammation, wrinkle fighters such as retinol, and a nonirritating sunscreen to protect this thin skin from UV radiation. It also may contain ingredients that reflect light to help minimize the appearance of dark circles and under-eye bags. Apply eye creams around the eye along the edge of the bone that outlines the eye socket.

For stretch marks: Few people, women especially, escape living without a few stretch marks. They are incredibly common among growing teens and pregnant women. In fact, about 70 percent of women get their first set in their teens from growth spurts; changes in breast size and fluctuations in weight also can cause new marks to form. Women in their thirties can have marks left over from their teens, and acquire more with pregnancy. If you have children later in life, your skin is less resilient and makes less collagen, so it doesn't bounce back as easily. Keeping the affected area supple and moisturized will go a long way to help mask the marks, as can self-tanners and waterproof makeup. If you're unhappy about the appearance of your marks and prefer to go the more invasive route, a series of laser treatments can help to minimize them.

For cellulite: Alongside stretch marks, cellulite ranks high on women's list of most stubborn beauty problems. The good news: the essence of the Water Secret will help you to reduce cellulite. Lumpy, textured skin affects 90 percent of women who have gone through puberty. Fad diets and fad formulas don't work to get rid of it, as most women know from experience. Contrary to what you may think, cellulite is not the result of too much fat in your body. It's caused by skin that has deteriorated to the point that buoyant fat cells are able to push into the middle layer of skin, the dermis, and show through the surface. By simply adding key skin-hydrating, cell-fortifying nutrients to your diet (the essence of the Water Secret), you can repair, rehydrate, and revitalize your skin to force stubborn fat cells back below the surface, where they are invisible—and keep them there. For more about treating cellulite, see my book *The Cellulite Solution: A Doctor's Program for Losing Lumps, Bumps, Dimples, and Stretch Marks*.

The Power and Promise in Peptides

As dermatologists, chemists, and manufacturers continued searching for new ways to address free radicals, cell renewal, inflammation, and hydration, the next milestone after the discovery of skin-specific antioxidants was the discovery of peptides.

Peptides, which are short chains of amino acids, have been touted to reduce wrinkles and skin roughness, among other things. They help increase the communication between skin cells so they can do what they're supposed to, more efficiently. It helps to think of them as messengers within cells, delivering commands that switch various functions on or off. Research has shown that we can use peptide technology to stimulate cells to increase the rate of skin cell regeneration and restore skin's ability to renew itself. We also may be able to literally turn on collagen production using peptides, but this area is still under investigation. Some peptides can be too large to penetrate deeply enough into the skin to be effective, but interest continues to be extremely high with peptides, and this is an ever-expanding category of ingredients. Studies are ongoing, but there is no doubt that many more peptides will be discovered in the near future. I encourage you to try products that have peptides in them to see how they make you look and feel.

Why Are Mushrooms and Licorice in My Face Cream?

The latest beauty craze has been coming from the kitchen, and it's not a marketing ploy. The more scientists dig deeper into natural ingredients for treating and nourishing the skin, the more they uncover about the healing powers of certain foods that can work wonders when incorporated into topical products. You can treat fine lines, sunburns, dullness, and splotches with ingredients you might not expect. Dietary substances known to be good for the complexion are sometimes better applied topically than ingested. As with vitamin C, you can get higher concentrations of ingredients in the skin by smoothing it directly onto the skin rather than ingesting them. This is why I'm a proponent of "feed your face." Here's a list of some of these exciting foods that can do just that when added to topicals:

- **Mushrooms:** All mushrooms are chock-full of compounds such as lipids, proteins, amino acids, and vitamins. They have strong antioxidant properties and may inhibit tumor growth. Mushrooms can help prevent the breakdown of collagen and elastin, thus keeping your skin firm and plump.
- **Apples:** Phloretin is a powerful antioxidant that comes only from the skin of an apple. It's one of the few that can be absorbed into the skin, neutralizing a large number of free radicals and reducing inflammation and hyperpigmentation.
- **Pomegranate:** I've been a huge fan of this fruit for years, and pioneered studies about its antiaging properties.

Pomegranate extracts have been used in facial products for years as a powerful antioxidant. We now believe that the extract may help decrease redness caused by sunburn. It's a triple benefit: products that contain pomegranate can help protect your skin from sun, increase the efficacy of sunscreen, and reduce redness if you do get a sunburn.

- **Durian:** Another secret weapon of mine is this tropical fruit, which grows in hot, humid climates. People eat durian because its sugars attract water into the cells, helping to maintain better hydration within the body. When applied topically, the skin remains hydrated longer because the moisture is continually being drawn to the cells. People with very dry skin would do well to seek a product with durian. You'll not only retain much-needed moisture more easily, but also that super-hydration will plump up your skin cells so the skin looks less wrinkly.
- **Licorice:** Licorice has long been thought to have an inhibiting effect on the creation of melanin, which is the coloring pigment in skin. You'll find it in products to treat hyperpigmentation. But now there's more reason to praise licorice for treating conditions such as psoriasis and dermatitis. Recent research shows that it can help greatly reduce inflammation as well as have anticancer effects.

Feeding Your Face Every Day: How to Create Your Personalized Skin Care Regimen

So what exactly should you be doing every day, and in which order? I've given you a number of ingredients to look for, which may have confused you about what your protocol should be on a daily or a weekly basis. Everything you do to meet your daily skin care needs should contain the appropriate ingredients, and above all, be simple and quick. You want to cleanse your skin, treat it with antiaging products, moisturize it, and protect it with sunscreen. If you have special concerns such as acne, discoloration, or advanced aging, you will need to make some slight modifications.

Here's the 411 on skin care, step by step:

1. *Gentle cleanser:* Wash your face twice a day with a gentle cleanser. This will remove dirt, debris, makeup, flakes of dead skin cells, and accumulated oils. Choosing a cleanser is a trial-and-error process. If your face feels dry, taut, and stiff thirty minutes after a wash, the cleanser is too harsh and you should try another one. Your skin should feel soft and pliable half an hour after you wash your face. A cleanser with hydroxy acids such as glycolic and salicylic acids is useful for most people because they exfoliate the skin during the cleansing and enhance hydration. Depending on your skin type, you may want to use an AHA/BHA skin cleanser every day, twice weekly, or just once a week. If you are prone to acne, you'll find cleansers designated for acne that contain special ingredients (notably benzoyl peroxide and/or salicylic acid) to help clear bacteria on the skin's surface that can lead to breakouts. Make sure to wash your face with warm—not hot—water. If you find benzoyl peroxide too drying and irritating, keep to just salicylic acid and be sure to moisturize. Don't be afraid to moisturize skin even though you have acne. It won't worsen it, and may, in fact, help to treat it.
2. *Toner:* Applied to freshly washed skin, toners help return the skin to a slightly acidic pH, where skin functions best. The protective layer on your skin that helps cripple growing bacteria and fungi while holding moisture in prefers an acidic environment. Most cleansers leave skin slightly on the alkaline (basic) side, which can make you more vulnerable to damage and infection. Even though your skin will naturally go back to a slightly acidic state, toners are refreshing, hydrating, and prep the skin for your moisturizer. If you choose to use one, make sure it's not too drying (some use harsh alcohols that can dry you out), and ideally find a toner that contains skin-soothing botanicals such as mint, cornflower, chamomile, or

bitter orange. Some toners also contain hydrating ingredients such as sodium PCA and/or amino acids. Those with antioxidants such as vitamin C and E offer an added bonus.

3. *Treat and repair:* If you are using any special formulas, such as retinoids, antioxidant infusions, or solutions for hyperpigmentation, you'd apply those before applying your moisturizer. Follow the instructions that come with the packaging. Some are best used at night, or both morning and night.
4. *Moisturize:* Again, always use a facial moisturizer with sunscreen in the morning, but at night switch to a thicker, sunscreen-free formula loaded with rich hydrators, antioxidants, and plant extracts. Don't worry about doubling up on ingredients such as antioxidants and skin soothers if they are in your treat-and-repair formulas as well as your moisturizer. You never can get enough of these antiaging miracles. You also may find a night formula that contains retinols, and that's okay, too. If you use a prescription-strength retinoid such as Retin-A, however, skip the night creams with added reintols.

Sometimes I get asked why it's necessary to go through this routine every single day. It's like brushing your teeth. If you skip a day, or two, or three, you've got lots of buildup to deal with, and you're not likely to get it all with one clean sweep. Wait too long to brush those pearly whites and you're likely to suffer from dental decay and inflamed gums, similar to breaking out on your face and seeing your pores clog up. It's not a pretty sight. So it really does pay to take care of your skin, every . . . single . . . day. (Your teeth, too.)

You don't need a separate makeup remover. A good cleanser can do the job without leaving leftover makeup. If you use heavy, waterproof makeup, however, you may choose to use a makeup remover in the areas where you need it.

As for exfoliating, that's a personal choice based on how sensitive your skin is and what you can tolerate. As often as your skin can take it is best. It's the difference between cleaning a floor routinely versus hiring a professional cleaning crew after it's been left alone too long and becomes a gunky mess. If you use a light exfoliant such as a hydroxy-acid wash, you should be able to exfoliate a few times a week. Go for the heavier-duty exfoliants, such as getting a facial or microdermabrasion, a few times a year.

Seeing a Dermatologist or Getting a Professional Facial

You'll want to visit a dermatologist once a year for a routine checkup and to address any specific concerns you have that you cannot seem to solve on your own. I recommend, however, that once you reach your thirties, scheduling visits a few times a year to a trained aesthetician (who can be working within a dermatologist's office or a spa) equipped to deliver pharmaceutical-grade treatments can be an excellent part of your wellness plan. Your particular skin needs will determine how frequently you go and which level of treatment you get.

Hassles with Hair Loss

Excessive hair loss affects 40 percent of women and 65 percent of men. While genetics do play a large role in how much hair we have, other factors could be going on. Your doctor can test to see if you are anemic, have low iron, or have an underperforming thyroid. Other medication you may be taking and stress also can be partly to blame. Most people don't have an underlying medical condition when their hair thins. A combination of hair-losing genes and stress is typically at play. Hair follicles are very sensitive to stress hormones, which explains why acute stress can bring on sudden hair loss, as the stress literally shocks hair follicles into an inactive state, after which they fall out. Once the follicle enters this resting phase prematurely, it stays there for about three months, after which time a large amount of hair will be shed. At any given time, a random number of hairs will be in various stages of growth and shedding. Pregnant women may notice thicker and healthier hair during their pregnancy, caused by the increased levels of hormones estrogen and progesterone, but after the baby is born, those hormone levels drop rapidly, triggering a shift from active to resting phases in the follicles. This explains why 20 to 45 percent of new moms may experience sudden hair loss about three months after giving birth. Most moms regain that hair within a year.

Assuming any underlying medical conditions are treated that could be causing thin hair or hair loss, the best way to treat your scalp and hair is to do what you'd do to your skin: routinely cleanse, nourish, and hydrate to ensure that the proper environment exists for healthy hair to grow and develop. You'll already be nourishing your hair from the inside out with the Cellular Water Secret Diet, and all you have to do is complement that regimen with shampoos and conditioners that don't contain harsh chemicals or overly dry out your hair. Ingredients I like to see in shampoos are natural plant extracts such as pomegranate and artemia; saw palmetto, which removes or blocks DHT—dihydrotestosterone, a natural metabolite of the body that causes hair loss; hyroxy acids to help ingredients penetrate the scalp; and phytantriol, which is vitamin B_5, to moisturize and protect hair.

Do Skin Types Matter?

There's no dearth of skin products on the market to match every skin type, but don't let it drive you crazy. Go by how your skin feels in response to the products you choose. Most people are oily in some places and drier in others. A few tips to consider:

- If you've got oily skin, don't be afraid to cleanse, treat, and moisturize twice a day, as would a person with dry skin. Even though your skin looks "moist" doesn't mean you couldn't be missing key lipids to maintain your skin's barrier. Your oil glands within the follicles are simply genetically programmed to be more active. Try a using cleanser with hydroxy acids on alternate days, or more often if your skin seems to respond well to it.
- Dry skin is the most fragile. Be careful about overcleansing and overexfoliating, as your skin is more susceptible to irritation. Use a cleanser and toner with hydrating ingredients and exfoliate gently (and not every day). Look for products that contain skin soothers such as chamomile extract and arnica.
- Fair-skinned people and those who spend a lot of time outdoors need to be extra cautious about overexposure to UV radiation. While a sunscreen with SPF 15 is sufficient for many, I recommend upping that coverage to at least 30 if you're more sensitive to the sun. Similarly, if you take drugs that increase your sensitivity to the sun, which is the case for birth control pills, for example, apply a broad-spectrum sunscreen with at least SPF 30.
- Don't overdo it. No matter what kind of skin you have, it's easy to overclean and overexfoliate and, in a word, irritate. You also can trigger excessive oil production with excessive use of soaps, cleansers, scrubs, and toners made with drying alcohols (some alcohols actually can be hydrating—there's a difference). Listen to what your skin is telling you and adjust your skin care routine accordingly.

> Pore size is genetically determined and unchangeable. You can, however, remove some of the debris that stretches the pores and makes them appear larger.

- Give products up to six months to work and show results.

What about Men?

Men typically don't pamper their faces the same way women do. The act of shaving, however, exfoliates their face. Many companies, including my own, design products especially for men that take into consideration the differences between male and female skin. And there are several differences. A quick rundown:

- *Smaller oil glands but more oil:* Men tend to have smaller oil glands, but they produce more oil due to higher levels of testosterone. After about age fifty, as hormonal aging kicks in stronger, oil production slows and a man's oil production is closer to that of a woman's.
- *Thicker but more irritable:* A man's skin is thicker than a woman's, which explains why women seems to show more signs of aging in their thinner (and more vulnerable) skin; but because most men shave every day, they scrape away a thin layer of lubricating film on the outermost part of the face. This can leave their skin more sensitive to irritants, and in general men are more exposed to damaging environmental elements than women are.
- *Older but better-looking:* If you've ever thought that men's skin seems to age better than women's, there's some truth to that. If a man and a woman are exposed to the same amount of sun in their lives, the man won't look as old as the woman even if they are the same age. Men don't lose the same amount of collagen as women do with age. A man's skin will thin, but the color and texture of a woman's face change more dramatically over time.

Men who are not accustomed to a daily skin care routine other than shaving are usually not inclined to start one, but they would do well to consider taking better care of their skin with topicals designed just for them. While they don't like to admit it, men do want their skin to look good. A daily cleanser and a moisturizer with sunscreen can help to prevent the same age-related skin issues that women are concerned about.

Most of the male patients I see come to me with specific problems, such as acne or a questionable mole, but once I treat their specific concern, I teach them how they can better protect their skin. As with Jacob in chapter 5, some of these patients return later to share incredible stories of transformation. Once they began to take care of their skin, they noticed results, which then inspired them to take care of other areas in their lives, such as diet and fitness. When you look better, you feel better about yourself and are more motivated to make further modifications in your lifestyle that can have a huge payoff. That's the whole point of the Water Secret. You don't have to change your entire life overnight. A single change, even just a slight shift in your daily skin care routine, can eventually add up to make a big impact.

A Note about Vitamin D

There's no longer a debate about the growing vitamin D deficiency in the general population. It's not just a result of people working indoors all day and protecting themselves from the sun's damaging rays, but it's also a consequence of geography. The vast majority of people who live in North America can't get the same amount of sunlight as those closer to the equator. It's easy for the body to manufacture plenty of vitamin D from brief exposure to UVB radiation a few times a week, but it's very hard to get that same amount of vitamin D from diet alone. Why is this vitamin so important? It's a hormone critical to survival, as a number of studies have found that higher levels of vitamin D, which the body makes when sunlight hits the skin, protects against some cancers and illnesses such as rickets, bone-thinning osteoporosis, and diabetes. It also helps the body's immune system work properly, reduces inflammation, and plays a role in muscle, cardiac, immune, and neurological functions.

That said, overexposure to UVB radiation is one of the leading causes of environmental aging, which shows up visibly on

In Their Own Words

I wanted to let you know what a difference Dr. Murad has had in my skin, hair, and nails. I was thrilled when Dr. Murad suggested placing me in a study. Prior to my visit with him, I had been to Botox parties where the emphasis was on quick injections without any discussion of skin care or healthy living. After I was placed in Dr. Murad's study and began treating my skin daily, the difference in my skin was very noticeable. People began to comment on how healthy my skin looked. I stopped wearing foundation because I didn't need it. My skin had a healthy glow. I took supplements faithfully and began to notice that my hair was thicker, shinier, and grew faster. My nails grew stronger, and the dimpling on my thighs lessened. I began to follow his Water Secret to the T and have lost about eight pounds. I will always be grateful for the chance to learn, after all these years, the proper way to take care of my skin and body. Thanks again for helping me look my best.

—Marilyn, forty

the skin. If you're not casually exposed to sunlight for brief periods a few days a week ("brief" meaning ten to fifteen minutes and long before you'd begin to burn), consider adding a vitamin D supplement that has at least 1,000 International Units to your daily regimen. Current recommendations for dosage of vitamin D supplements (400 IU) have been proven to be inadequate. I do, however, think it's important to keep your face protected; it is always exposed and is the most prominent place to show accelerated aging.

To Cut, Slice, Burn . . . or Not

Deciding whether or not to take a more aggressive approach to enhance your appearance is a personal decision, and one that can take some soul-searching. Going into detail about every option available to you is beyond the scope of this book. I encourage you to find and consult with a trusted doctor in your area so you can have a real conversation about what you may or may not want to consider. There is an array of cosmetic medical procedures today, from noninvasive laser skin treatments to high-tech skin rejuvenation procedures that entail some downtime and discomfort.

Regardless of your decision to incorporate these techniques into your life, following the Water Secret will complement their results and give you a "face-lift." I'll admit that I'm a big advocate for the medical-spa industry—antiaging centers like my own that offer a menu of services from basic spa treatments to medical procedures performed by physicians. I wholeheartedly believe that these will become the health centers of the future—places where people can go to get customized attention and care. They also afford us something largely missing from our lives today and sorely needed: time to relax, unwind, and remove ourselves from the daily grind that increasingly pushes our limits of being able to cope with stress.

Stress gets a lot of ink in media circles, but one type of stress that's relatively new to us as a people and a society is what I call Cultural Stress. I've already mentioned Cultural Stress a few times so far, but I've saved it for a comprehensive discussion for last. Why? Because it's among the most pervasive hallmarks of everyday life that can tie a big knot in your attempts to live a healthy life. Remember, taking care of your emotional health constitutes the third prong to Inclusive Health alongside caring for your internal and external cellular health, and that's where Cultural Stress resides. You'll need every tip I've already given you to this point to address Cultural Stress and knock it down. Although it may seem to be an intangible and invisible behemoth, Cultural Stress sneakily zooms in on cells and wrings them dry without you necessarily feeling or noticing it at first. Its effects, however, are cumulative and emerge over time. The good news is that managing Cultural Stress is highly possible, even when regular stress is here to stay.

CHAPTER 8

Combat Cultural Stress

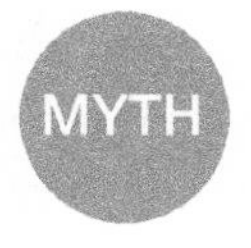

Modern stress is unavoidable.

It's 1:20, and Susan, a longtime friend, is late for lunch with you. She rushes in, drops her belongings, and collapses in her chair, declaring, "It's been a crazy day, so sorry I'm late." You tell her no problem, that you're glad to see her, but part of you worries that you'll be late getting back to work by two in time to meet a deadline and then pick up the kids promptly at three. Just when you dive into conversation as Susan looks at the menu, her cell phone rings. She looks at it briefly and then turns it off. You begin again.

When the waiter comes to take your orders, you sneak a peek at your BlackBerry to check in with your son's teacher (you recalled his report card was going to be e-mailed to you by one o'clock). You open it, gasp at the grades, and think—How can he get into college with these marks? Your heartbeat accelerates. You're distracted. All you can think about is finishing your lunch so you can call the school and perhaps set a time to talk to the teacher later that day. In the meantime, another e-mail comes in, from the bank, alerting you to your overdrawn account, and then another message drops in, from a colleague at work, announcing an emergency on the very project you were going to take care of back at the office.

Your head begins to spin. Suddenly everything seems urgent and important and you can't handle it all in one fell swoop. "PLS RETRN NOW!" reads another message, this one from your boss. You look up at your friend, apologize, and then frantically think about what to do next. Bail on lunch? Call the school? The office? The bank? Who gets your attention first? You can feel the sweat start pumping.

Welcome to the cult of Cultural Stress. Surely you can relate to part of this scenario. Just reading this may have stressed you out!

When was the last time you made someone laugh? Or booked a massage? Played hooky from work to play with friends in town? Had lunch with someone and truly lost all sense of time and felt really *happy*, like a kid in a candy store?

If you're still thinking about those times, if they ever existed, then it has been too long.

My patients inspire me every day. Many of them are suffering way beyond the skin condition that brought them to my examining room. One woman I'll call Michelle was suffering from psoriasis, which is a crusty and itchy disease that can flare up under stressful situations. When I asked Michelle about her stress, she confided that her family caused her much stress. She hadn't spoken to her parents for more than a year, she was estranged from her sister, and she was having occasional spats with her husband that disturbed her.

As part of her medical exam I tested her cellular water levels and, sure enough, she was very low. Her system was depleted. I talked to Michelle about her diet, her exercise, and her emotional well-being. I explained that trying to deal with her communication with her family would be an adjunct to the salves and internal treatments I would be prescribing. I also suggested that she might see a psychologist or family therapist to help with those emotional stresses if she couldn't do it alone. Michelle was a wonderful listener, but I wasn't confident that she'd take action. But she did. Before she returned for her six-week checkup, she called me to relate the story of reconnecting with her sister after talking to a therapist. When she told a similar story about her relationship with her husband, she was so happy that she began to cry. Michelle realized that she had been so tightly wound up in her problems that she'd forgotten to turn to her husband and simply talk to him.

I share this story because Michelle is not alone. It's very easy to forget (read "avoid") to communicate with the people we love. It's also very easy to let what I call Cultural Stress invade our lives. We're busy. We're multitasking. We're commuting. We're obsessively checking our retirement portfolios. We're trying to keep up with ourselves and our racetrack culture at the expense of health and genuine happiness.

In recent studies of the so-called blue zones—places where people live long, lean lives well into their nineties and beyond—the common denominator is clear: a low-stress lifestyle. They maintain a positive outlook on life, belong to a tightly knit community, and keep family first. They move naturally in everyday life, consume fresh local ingredients, and processed food is not part of their daily diet. One zone in particular—the only blue zone in the United States—is a stone's throw away from the densely populated, smoggy city of Los Angeles. This community, of Seventh-Day Adventists in Loma Linda, California, defies the stereotype that you have to live like a hermit in a pristine, remote area to avoid a short life. Another group, in Sardinia, Italy, is comprised of sheepherders who spend their days walking, enjoying family and friends routinely, and drinking local red wine with their meals. The famous Okinawan residents of Japan drink mugwort sake, remain active, and honor the elderly. In short, these people live by the tenets of the Water Secret without knowing it. Masters of healthy living, they may not know what stress is, at least not in the same way the average American does.

Emotional care is sorely neglected in our society, yet emotions create a strong and powerful undercurrent to our health. The role of modern medicine is so focused on acute disease that we forget to ask ourselves, "What is true health?"

The world in which we live is not only causing us to feel time-deprived and anxious, but also the resultant stress is adding tremendous pressure on our biological systems.

This is when we can turn to unhealthy habits that push us in a wrong direction and leave us ever more tired, uncreative, drug- and stimulant-dependent, and unsatisfied. During the course of my work with more than fifty thousand patients, I've discovered that using the Water Secret to create healthy, hydrated cells helps the body fight aging and disease and, most importantly, the ruinous effects of Cultural Stress. Since coining this new type of stress, I've prompted a new field of studies now under way to investigate just how influential Cultural Stress is on health and wellness, and what we can do about its negative consequences. Unbeknownst to many, Cultural Stress is unlike traditional forms of stress critical to survival. Cultural Stress is wholly unnecessary for survival, yet today it is pervasive, and its effects are cumulative.

Cultural stressors are not limited to work, bosses, kids, tardiness, technostress, and incessant e-mail. We experience other factors from the environment that compound daily Cultural Stress levels, including pollution, droughts, and worries about access to safe drinking water. According to the second UN World Water Development Report, more than a billion people—almost a fifth of the world's population—lack access to safe drinking water, and 40 percent lack access to basic sanitation. The United Nations estimates that by 2050, more than two billion people in forty-eight countries will lack sufficient water. Drought conditions can cause a vast number of devastating conditions that will affect everyone as the prices for goods and services increase. When food crops and grass and grain used to feed livestock and poultry suffer, our groceries will become more expensive. In addition, drought conditions can lead to a wide range of life-threatening diseases, wildfires, social or political conflict, war, migration, or relocation. The list goes on and on.

We are ill adapted to handle this kind of stress, and it could very well be what brings the average life span down for the first time in modern history—rolling back the gains brought by advancements in medicine and technology.

The good news is that Cultural Stress is largely manageable. But before we get to those stress antidotes, let's look at what stress means and how it physically affects all of us the same, regardless of the specific stressor.

Being truly healthy does not only mean the body is free of diabetes, cancer, or other afflictions; being healthy also involves a passion for life, a true connection with others, and an overall positive sense of self.

The Science of Stress: Why It Feels So beyond Your Control

The second you were born was probably the first time you really felt stress, and you probably cried. We've all experienced myriad stressful situations since birth. What stresses you out? Money? Health? Kids? Fear of failure? Perhaps success stresses you out. Ask the question a thousand times and you'll get a thousand different answers. What's clear is that from birth, we live with stress. And today it's become clear that stress is directly linked to the six leading causes of death in the United States, including heart disease, cancer, accidents, and suicide.

What Is Stress?

Most of us can recognize the symptoms of stress. We feel it. We become irritable, our heart races, our face feels hot, we feel the familiar headache or upset stomach, suddenly our deodorant seems to have lost its power as wetness builds, there's a feeling of impending doom, and we're irritated by the smallest things. For some people, stress has little outward effect. For these individuals, what they feel at the surface is internalized and sometimes expressed as depression or disease. In fact, many of these people don't believe they experience stress, but they do; they just don't consciously recognize it until it builds up to a certain point and seeps out in other ways.

The term *stress*, as it is used today, was coined in 1936 by one of the founding fathers of stress research, Hans Selye, who defined it as "the nonspecific response of the body to any demand for change." Essentially, Selye proposed that when subjected to persistent stress, both humans and animals could develop certain life-threatening afflictions, such as heart attacks and strokes, which were thought to be caused by specific pathogens only. This is a crucial point because it illuminates the impact that everyday life and experiences have not only on our emotional well-being but also on our physical health.

The word stress as it relates to emotions became part of our vocabulary in the 1950s. Its use became common with the onset of the Cold War, an era when fear ruled. We were frightened of atomic war, so we built bomb shelters. As a society, we could not say we were "afraid"; instead we used the word stress. Today we continue to use the word to describe anything that disrupts us emotionally—we're stressed, stressed out, under stress, and so on. Stress also can be described as the thoughts, feelings, behaviors, and physiological changes that happen when we respond to demands and perceptions. And if those demands placed on us overwhelm our perceived ability to cope, we experience stress. We begin to pant silently in our frenzied minds like an animal, probably looking for an escape, too.

Giving a Public Speech Is Not the Same as Giving Your Kids a Lecture

Since Selye, researchers have broken down stress into several subcategories. Stress physiology has come a long way in particular in the past fifty years, and so have the stressors. One hundred years ago people worried about dying from influenza, polio, or giving birth. Now we worry about the illnesses that are likely to creep up on us as we get older and more worn out physically. Those illnesses include the most common killers of today: heart disease, cancer, and stroke. Rather than striking us suddenly like a crouching tiger, these diseases slowly build up over time, gathering strength based on our lifestyles until they finally emerge and either dim our lights or shut them off completely.

Clinically, we now categorize stress in three ways: acute stress, episodic acute stress, and chronic stress.

Acute stress is short-term and is the most common form of stress. This type of stress comes from things such as taking a test, giving a speech, or avoiding an accident. Once the test, speech, or threat of an accident is over, the stress goes away. Your body's physical reaction to the stress also wanes, which I'll get to shortly. Acute stress is the most treatable and manageable kind of stress (because it's over pretty quickly!). It's also probably the most ancient form of stress because it's what got us out of life-threatening situations when we were roaming the savanna among wild animals. Millennia ago, threats to our livelihood were more clear-cut, and we relied on the famous flight-or-fight response to leap out of harm's way. But over the past several hundred years we've moved out of the real jungle and into a new one of our own making. These days, stress is more likely to come at us from modern aggravations and responsibilities: the stress of hearing chronically bad news, driving in commuter traffic, juggling tight finances, and so on. Unlike a brief encounter with a wild animal—an encounter you either win or lose in seconds—modern stress can often be relentless, and the effects are cumulative.

Episodic acute stress happens to those who live in chaos. Those who experience this kind of stress seem always to be rushing, but ironically, they're habitually late. They are supremely busy but don't necessarily get a single thing accomplished on time. Or they don't finish projects because they frantically move from one task to another ad nauseam. We all know people who fall into this category.

Chronic stress is the worst kind and can be debilitating. This is the stress that people feel when they cannot see a way out of a miserable situation, and there are plenty of examples here: an unhappy marriage, an ongoing struggle with your (teenage) kids, a serious health challenge, debt, poverty, a horrible job, or no job at all. The economic events of the past few years have led to an epidemic of chronic stress in our world. Those who experience chronic stress tend to lack solid coping skills, and rather than have optimistic outlooks on life no matter what's going on, they ruminate in the past, worry about the future, and generally see the glass as half empty all the time. They hold on to their pessimistic attitude like a blanket, even though it does them more harm than good.

While these three categories have been adequate for the past several decades, so much has changed in the years since *stress* first entered our dictionaries. It's become necessary to add Cultural Stress.

A New Stress Sending Us over the Edge

Cultural Stress is a new type of stress that is superimposed on the normal stresses of everyday life. It began infiltrating our lives as we became more technologically savvy and affluent. Technology now allows us to work and communicate anywhere, anytime, twenty-four hours a day, and this makes America a land of a constantly logged-on workforce. According to a U.S. government report, Americans work longer hours than nearly anyone in the developed world—even the Japanese. For many professionals, the forty-hour workweek doesn't exist anymore. Sixty-to-eighty-hour workweeks are now the norm. We have voice mail, e-mail, texting, paging, and are still bombarded with paper snail mail. From the advent of the digital revolution in the 1980s, to increased population and affluence, to the world-changing events on September 11, 2001, to the recent climate of unending economic anxiety, many of life's stressors have taken a more prominent and invasive position in our daily lives.

Cultural Stress is like a ceaseless refrigerator hum rather than an infrequent phone ring. Another perfect example of Cultural Stress is traffic congestion. No matter where you go, it seems that traffic only gets worse. The anxiety, frustration, fear, and reflexes you need to drive defensively to get from point A to point B on time add a considerable amount of Cultural Stress to everyday living. Traffic and driving time must always be considered with daily schedules, and these thought processes add Cultural Stress to everything we do. On the other hand, a minor fender bender is a stand-alone event, and an example of basic acute (and sometimes episodic if you experience it on occasion) stress.

Signs of Cultural Stress are apparent even in infants and young children. One study reported in *Skin and Allergy News*, showed that infants living within a hundred meters of stop-and-go traffic experienced a 2.5-fold increase of noncold wheezing than those living more than a hundred meters away. These infants experienced constant traffic, noise, and air pollution, which were indicated as prime contributors to the babies' Cultural Stress levels.

Stressed Out at Work, and on the Way to Work

According to the federal government's National Institute for Occupational Safety and Health, 40 percent of workers find their jobs stressful, and 75 percent of people surveyed believe their jobs are more stressful now than a generation ago. Nearly 3.5 million Americans spend an hour and a half or more each way to work and back. Commuters are filling 4:00 A.M. trains into major cities, and restaurants that opened for breakfast at 6 are opening earlier to accommodate the bleary-eyed workforce. But you probably already knew this. You know it because you live it. And you're not alone.

Depressing fact: The World Health Organization has estimated that by the year 2020, depression will be the second-leading disability-causing disease in the world. In many developed countries, such as the United States, depression is already among the top causes in terms of disability and excess mortality.

You would think that with all of this overworking, we'd be more productive. To a certain extent we are. But there's a limit to the productivity. While it's true that stress stimulates a high level of performance, there's a threshold where performance begins to progressively degrade and negatively affect our output and creativity. It's the classic law of diminishing returns.

Americans in Isolation

Cultural Stress, whether caused by fear, overwork, or too many options causing conflict in decision-making, ultimately leads to isolation. I believe isolation to be one of the most prominent diseases in today's world. Studies have shown that to

The Culprits of Cultural Stress

- Cell phones, wireless Internet, and handheld computers are used anywhere, anytime, 24-7. *Information overload*.
- People are working longer hours than ever. *Work overload*.
- Rush hours are starting earlier and ending later. Work travel replaces family time. *Isolation overload*.
- Nearly half of working mothers are heavily stressed every day. It takes a village to raise children, but many parents are doing it solo.
- Today's family is increasingly isolated as the stress of modern life pushes them apart.
- Even young children are suffering from anxiety due to Cultural Stress.

reduce isolation, people need to have regular physical and social contact, which reduces Cultural Stress and leads to happier, healthier lives. In my own studies, I've found that the water content of patients who are around others is higher than those who isolate themselves, or who don't realize they isolate themselves until they describe their daily rituals of driving to and from work alone, and working in a cubicle all day. This is a modern form of torture. Think about it: what do they do with prisoners who misbehave? They place them in isolation. As highly social, emotional beings, being isolated is distressing.

And even though we like to think we live in a very connected society now thanks to e-mail and texting, for example, these very devices can worsen feelings of isolation. We sit and type rather than listen to someone's voice on the phone. We blog about what's going on in our lives to strangers and forget to gather around our nearest and dearest for dinner in person to catch up. There is no substitute for human contact and authentic interactions that don't entail spell-checks and links to scripted videos. Real life is never scripted.

It Starts Early

Cultural Stress starts young. And while parents may not like to hear this, they are the ones who initiate it in their children.

Of Mice and Men

New research in mice suggests that social isolation may promote more damaging inflammation in the brain during a stroke. Researchers found that all the male mice that lived with a female partner survived seven days after a stroke, but only 40 percent of socially isolated animals lived that long. This doesn't mean you have to live with a spouse or a partner; you just have to routinely connect with others and stay connected. Had the coupled mice had cell phones and computers to interact, I'm not sure if that would have had the same impact.

Traffic Jam in Your Heart

New research from Germany shows that people who had heart attacks were three times more likely than not to have been sitting in traffic an hour before their symptoms began. And for some strange reason not identified yet, a woman's risk of heart attack is five times higher within an hour of being in traffic than that of women not in traffic.

New parents are often anxious about getting their child into the best preschool. In fact, it's common for unborn children to be placed on a preschool wait list. The next focus is on ensuring that the child is enrolled in all the right extracurricular activities—from preschool through high school. This cycle puts pressure on children to excel at a very young age, while placing a burden on the parents to make more money to pay for the education and the extracurricular activities. No wonder parents are under enormous stress today.

This scenario, coupled with our society's increasing financial troubles, has a far-reaching domino effect. To make more money to pay for living expenses, we are working longer hours. We are accepting an unprecedented level of stress in our lives. All of this has put a great strain on our health and well-being, especially because the vast majority of Americans are barely keeping up.

So it's not surprising that over the past few years doctors in all fields of medicine have seen a dramatic change in their patients' stress levels. Patients come in the office with their smart phones and iPods and they are telling their physicians how alone they feel, despite the fact that all these communication tools should keep them more connected.

The average American has about fifty brief stress attacks a day.

Anatomy of an Attack

From an evolutionary and survivalist perspective, stress is a good thing. It's supposed to prime the body for battle and get us out of harm's way. The problem, though, is that our physical reaction is the same every time we sense a potential threat, whether it's real and coming from something truly life-threatening, or just the to-do list and an overbearing boss.

First, the brain signals to the adrenal glands to release epinephrine, better known as adrenaline. This is what causes your heart to pick up speed as blood rushes to your muscles in case you need to make a run for it. That adrenaline, by the way, steals blood from the skin and face to allocate it toward your muscles, which is why you can suddenly look pale as a ghost or become "white with fear."

As soon as the threat passes, your body returns to normal. If the threat doesn't pass and your stress response gets stronger, then a whole wave of stress hormones gets released in a series of events known as the hypothalamic-pituitary-adrenal (HPA) axis. The hypothalamus, a region of the brain, first releases a stress coordinator called corticotropin-releasing hormone (CRH). CRH then delivers a message to a pea-sized gland at the base of your brain called the pituitary, telling it to release another hormone, called adrenocorticotropic hormone (ACTH). ACTH then moves through the bloodstream until it hits the adrenals, which then let cortisol loose.

Emotional Command Center

The hypothalamus is frequently referred to as the seat of our emotions. It's our chief leader in emotional processing. The split second you feel anxious, deeply worried, scared, or simply concerned that you can't pay a bill, the hypothalamus secretes the hormone CRH, which starts a domino effect ending in cortisol rushing into your bloodstream.

Surely you've heard about cortisol before. It's the body's chief stress hormone, aiding in that famous fight-or-flight response. It also controls how your body processes carbs, fats, and proteins, and helps it to reduce inflammation. Because it's the hormone responsible for protecting you, its actions increase your appetite, tell your body to stock up on more fat, and break down materials that can be used for quick forms of energy, including muscle. Not all what you'd like to happen, but when your body senses stress (even when you know it's not the kind that will physically kill you in ten seconds or less), it thinks you won't see food again for a while or it may need an ample supply of fuel to camp out on during a famine or use to make a mad dash. In other words, cortisol causes tissues to break down, including muscle, skin, and collagen, while at the same time assembling fat.

For this reason, excessive cortisol levels can wreak havoc on the body, making it hard to lose weight, replenish cells, encourage the growth of new cells, and form new youth-building collagen. Everything takes a hit, including blood vessels that become more fragile and can't keep meeting the demands. As cells lose their capacity to hold on to moisture, they become less resilient. You begin to see this aging on your skin as lines get deeper and more visible on the surface. Imagine what's going on inside. Cellular turnover slows down considerably, and you dry out even faster.

Cortisol does, however, serve a positive role. It helps immune cells attack infectious invaders and tells the brain when those invaders have been taken care of. And another way to look at its effects in mobilizing fat and upping your appetite is that it builds up energy reserves (calories) that your muscles may need soon. But for the most part, you don't need those energy reserves because you're not in dire straits. You're just overreacting to a trivial stressor that your body interprets as something serious. But it has a profound impact on you regardless.

Emotional Attachments

I constantly find myself drilling the same message into patients when I explain to them that the skin is connected to their emotions. For centuries, ancient medical practices and cultures have appreciated the connections between mind and body in wellness and disease, yet conventional medicine still trivializes this complex set of relationships. Hopefully that will change, given recent evidence.

The scientific study of the impact of stress on the body from the inside out, and even the outside in, has made tremendous advances in the past decade. In 1998, doctors from Harvard University conducted a joint study with several Boston-area hospitals designed to examine the connections and interactions between the mind and the body, specifically the skin. They dubbed their findings the NICE network, which stands for neuro-immuno-cutaneous-endocrine. In plainspeak, it's a network consisting of your nervous system, immune system, the skin, and your endocrine (hormonal) system. All of these are intimately connected through a dialogue of shared interactive chemicals. Like a giant wireless network, when one phone rings, the others can hear it and respond.

These Boston researchers studied how various external forces affect our state of mind, from massage and aromatherapy to depression and isolation. What they discovered confirmed what we had already known anecdotally for centuries: our state of mind has a definite impact on our health and even our looks. People suffering from depression, for example, look older and less healthy, and not because they've "let themselves go" and aren't grooming themselves as rigorously as their happier counterparts. They actually are older than happier comrades who are the same biological age. The stress of living with depression has accelerated the aging process and damaged their health.

Another area of hot study in the past decade has been examining the skin's own stress-response system. Research indicated that the skin-centered response has an impact on par with the brain-centered HPA axis response. Skin doesn't just respond to the hormonal signals generated by the HPA axis response even though several hormones and neurotransmitters released inside the body have receptors in the skin. Our skin manages its own independent and fully functional system that acts very much like the hypothalamic-pituitary-adrenal axis. It can produce the same molecules locally, including CRH, ACTH, and cortisol. Just as your adrenal glands can release cortisol in a virtual instant, so, too, can pigment cells in your skin and hair follicles release stress hormones.

Skin also can manufacture beta-endorphins, serotonin, and melatonin, the last two of which are hormones key to mood. It's amazing to think that our skin has its own stress-response system and shares a common language with our nervous system. It not only responds to what our brains tell it, but the skin also can initiate responses and send messages through its own network. This helps explain how myriad psychological and physical (including excessive exposure to the sun's UV rays or a hot stove) stress triggers can have secondary consequences to our appearance and health. Colds become harder to fight, and skin disorders such as acne and eczema worsen.

> Cultural Stress is part of life. It's something that affects all of us, but it doesn't have to take over our lives.

Cultural Stress and Your Health

Because the body responds to all forms and sources of stress the same, I think Cultural Stress is having a greater impact on the state of our health than most people realize. (If only our bodies were smart enough to save the stress response for real threats and ignore petty aggravations, we'd be a lot healthier. Maybe in another million years or so.)

In recent years I have observed an increase in rosacea and adult acne, which I believe are directly related to an increase in Cultural Stress. It's already been shown in research circles that stress can increase the production of certain hormones that worsen acne. One skin condition in particular that I believe may be attributed to Cultural Stress is an increase in facial hair among adult women, which can be embarrassing to the point of heartbreaking. There's nothing more frustrating than growing hair where it doesn't belong, or where you just don't want it, while at the same time losing hair in other places where you *do* want it. Hormonal shifts and the outpouring of androgens, namely testosterone, when you're stressed can cause you to lose hair (on your head, for example), and it also can cause hair to suddenly appear in places where it didn't previously exist (such on your face or chin).

The good news is that we can counteract Cultural Stress and improve our health both physically and emotionally with the Water Secret. Cultural Stress contributes to damaged cell membranes, which, in turn, allows the precious water that keeps them functioning to escape. We know that stress releases neuropeptides, for example, that directly damage cellular membranes. The resultant water loss, as you know by

In Their Own Words

I have always lived with the philosophy of connectedness. Life flows in and out of people and their environments, influencing and altering everything it touches. Yet, before knowing Dr. Murad, I never knew how to connect my skin with the rest of my life. I would isolate many parts of my body, treating them as segregated items. Learning how intertwined our emotional, internal, and external states are has brought not only my skin into balance, but my life as well. I've brought my breakouts to nonexistent by taking care of my face daily and reducing my stress. I've become more committed to yoga and my running routine. Bringing exercise back into my life has encouraged healthy, not diet-oriented, eating. By utilizing recipes from Dr. Murad, avoiding certain foods, and taking supplements, I've boosted my hydration levels, increased my energy levels, and upped my mood—all of which have helped defend against negative emotions and stress. Dr. Murad has gifted me with tools that have taken my skin and my life to an integrated health approach that I never would have been able to find on my own.

—Carrie H., fifty-five

now, has myriad effects. It causes our cells and connective tissue to break down, which prevents our heart, lungs, brain, and other organs from functioning at optimal levels—all of which become apparent when you look at the skin. I'm frequently astonished at how much a simple vacation can enhance patients' Phase Angle, indicating improvement in the strength of their cell membranes and cellular water retention.

Of course, there's more to removing stress from our lives than soaking in a fragrant bath, taking a vacation, or getting a massage. If it were that simple, then many of the stress-induced illnesses and afflictions that we see every day in our world would fade away. The best way to keep stress at bay is to learn how to manage it so it affects you less.

The Antidotes to Cultural Stress

If it's not personal, don't take it personally.

So how can you deal with all of this without moving to Pluto? For starters, being fully educated on different types of stress and their effects on you will help you take that initial step in managing them better. We're living in one of the most exciting times. So much good has come with all the technology and advances we've experienced. Scientifically, we're only just realizing the power of human emotion and its effects on all the body's systems, how it influences skin conditions, and its ability to magnify disease. It's easy to tell people to relax or to be good to themselves, but when stress is so pervasive that there's no hiding from or avoiding it, it takes effort to unplug.

The reality is that our lives will become even more digitized as time goes on, and we will continue to push our children and ourselves to capacity until we wear out. As Americans, it's not easy to unlearn the need to be on the go, but when it comes to mental and physical health, a day, a week, or a month of complete relaxation may be just what the doctor ordered. Everything in moderation is the key, and this includes the

Flushing Stress Out

The power of exercise in reducing stress is well known. But here's something you might not have known: Exercise makes your blood circulate more quickly, transporting the stress hormone (and fat-friendly) cortisol to your kidneys and flushing it out of your system. Remember, cortisol encourages your body to store fat—especially visceral fat—that releases fatty acids into your blood, raising cholesterol and insulin levels and paving the way for heart disease and diabetes. One study found that eighteen minutes of walking three times per week can quickly lower the hormone's levels by 15 percent.

things that contribute to Cultural Stress. The goal is to reduce Cultural Stress while enjoying the simple pleasures of life.

To that end, let me share some ideas to combat Cultural Stress. Other than the usual stress-reducing aspects you've already learned—regular exercise and a nutrient-rich diet—see how many of the following "gets" you can begin to incorporate into your life starting today.

Get a Hobby

The old advice *Get a life!* has some substance to it. When you get a hobby, it forces you to take time out for yourself and do something enjoyable, while providing time for you to reflect. Life seems more worthwhile and pleasurable. And you have reason to seek out others who share your enthusiasm for that hobby, opening the door to connect and relate more with others.

Happiness has gained a lot of attention in recent years, as volumes of books and studies have emerged to help explain what makes us happy, or not. One of the prevailing pieces of wisdom from the studies defines happiness as the pursuit of engaging and meaningful activities.

The Happiness Test

Which of the following would make you happier?

- Making more money
- Finding a soulmate
- Losing ten pounds
- Moving into a new house
- Success
- Better genes

Hard to answer? New science proves that happiness is a process, not a goal. And it's not necessarily about having "fun," either. Happiness is about 50 percent genetic, 40 percent intentional, and 10 percent circumstantial. That 40 percent category—the intentional one—is the most important. Circumstances can change or you can become accustomed to them (a new car, a bigger house, or a promotion, for example) such that they no longer make you "happy." On the other hand, when you are engaged in a life's purpose that has meaning to you, which can be anything from rearing children to doctoring the elderly in underserved areas, happiness finds you in the way you live and look at the world. In other words, happiness is more a choice than an outcome or a destination. It's an action, not a result.

Get Connected

The self-help and alternative medicine market is colossal, no doubt spurred by an increasing demand for clues to better health, more energy, and vibrant living. In search of that holy grail of health, however, many people overlook a powerful weapon that could help them fight illness and depression, speed recovery, slow aging, and prolong life: their friends. Researchers are only now starting to pay attention to the importance of friendship and social networks in overall health. A ten-year Australian study found that older people with a large circle of friends were 22 percent less likely to die during the study period than those with fewer friends. A large 2007 study showed an increase of nearly 60 percent in the risk for obesity among people whose friends gained weight. And in 2009, Harvard researchers reported that strong social ties could promote brain health as we age.

One of the easiest ways to reduce your isolation is to join a group that shares similar hobbies, philosophies, and interests. Get involved in community events. This can be any number of things. It can entail activities or involvements such as group exercise classes; professional groups or associations; book clubs; potluck dinner nights with friends; charity events at your kids' schools or your town hall; volunteering at a nearby Red Cross, hospital, YMCA chapter, or nonprofit; or signing up for a class at a local community college. There are so many ideas that I'd love for you to write me about what you've been up to. Opportunities abound in this department if you open yourself up to them.

Get Disconnected

There's a strange duality to being attached to machines that allow us to connect with others around the world in an instant. From cell phones to social networks that can transmit what you're doing right now in fractions of a second, communication these days is quick; easy; and, to a large degree, isolating. When you resort to electronic transmissions of information rather than speaking to someone in person or even over the phone, you lose a human touch to the experience. You also have a tendency to lose focus, as those transmissions become rapid-fire, frequent, distracting, and intrusive. I admire people who make a choice to carve out time once or twice a week when they put down their smart phones and don't check their e-mail. It can be incredibly invigorating and stress-reducing to disconnect yourself occasionally from the digital world. See if you can designate a single day a week, perhaps a whole weekend from time to time, when you let the voice mail and the e-mail pile up. Detach yourself from the need to keep checking and responding to the constant, chattering influx—much of which is not important, not urgent, and not helpful to your health and well-being.

Get Touched

I think everyone should visit a spa or a massage therapy center as frequently as possible. I know that for many it may seem like a luxury, but it doesn't have to be. If you were to add up the cost of eating dinner out once a week for a month, you'd have plenty of money to get a massage, body scrub, and/or facial and enjoy all the amenities offered at most spas. Instead of eating out, cook a homemade meal and invite friends over for dinner once a week. Add up those extra dollars and put them toward a monthly or bimonthly spa treatment. The healing power of touch is grossly underestimated in our society, yet it's one of the most potent tools for emotional care. Massage not only benefits the muscles and tissues being kneaded and stretched but also has been found to lower stress levels significantly. It's been shown to increase weight gain in premature infants, alleviate depression, reduce pain in cancer patients, improve sleep patterns, and positively alter the immune system. Research from the renowned Touch Research Institute shows that it's as beneficial to touch as it is to be touched. And, more recently, researchers at the University of North Carolina, alongside scientists in Europe, are unraveling how the body responds to pleasurable touch. They have identified a class of nerve fibers in the skin that specifically send pleasure messages. Called the C-tactile nerve fibers, they send feel-good messages to the brain upon stimulation through pleasurable touch.

Healing touch therapy can take many forms, not just classic massage. Experiment with what your local spa has to offer. Bring this concept to home and into the bedroom with your partner, too. In between the more elaborate spa visits, schedule brief, inexpensive manicures, pedicures, or simply exchange five minutes of chair massage with your best friend at work.

Studies have shown that these can dramatically reduce job stress while increasing productivity and alertness.

Get the Morning Off to a Good Start

Deficiencies in B vitamins, vitamin C, calcium, and magnesium stress out your body and trigger an increase in cortisol levels, not to mention food cravings. Too many people skip breakfast, and can easily find themselves lacking these critical nutrients. This can instigate a vicious cycle of eating poorly throughout the day, relying on caffeine to stay alert and productive, then turning to sleep aids at night to wind down. Start the day right with a nutrient-rich breakfast that contains vitamins, and not just the ones in your multivitamin.

Try a handful of berries (vitamin C), six to eight ounces of low-fat yogurt (calcium and magnesium), and a slice of whole-grain toast with natural peanut butter. Whole grains are loaded with B vitamins, while peanut butter contains fatty acids that can decrease the production of stress hormones. Peanut butter also will keep you satisfied longer.

Get Out of Your Box

Try something totally different from your normal routine. Take a yoga class. Test out a new sport. Go for a hike. Choose to do something you've never done before. It will challenge you in fresh ways, and inspire you to have a more positive outlook on life. Engaging in fun, novel activities can be surprisingly fulfilling and relaxing.

Get Deep with Your Breath

Slow, controlled breathing is the foundation for many Eastern practices such as yoga, qigong, tai chi, and classic meditation—all of which aim to plunge the body (and mind, clearly) into a balanced, stress-free state. One of the reasons why deep breathing is so helpful is that it triggers a parasympathetic nerve response, as opposed to a sympathetic nerve response, the latter of which is sensitive to stress and anxiety. At the onset of stress, the sympathetic nervous system springs into action and is largely responsible for those oft-damaging spikes in the stress hormones cortisol and adrenaline. The parasympathetic nervous system, on the other hand, can trigger a relaxation response, and deep breathing is the quickest means of getting these two systems to communicate. You can flip the switch from high alert to low in seconds as your heart rate slows, muscles relax, and blood pressure lowers.

Keep track of positive things that happened during the day and replay those in your mind when negative thoughts intrude. Or call a friend when your mind starts racing.

Deep breathing can be done anywhere, anytime. Sit comfortably in a chair or lie down.

Close your eyes and make sure your body is relaxed, releasing all tension in your neck, arms, legs, and back. Inhale through your nose for as long as you can, feeling your diaphragm and abdomen rise as your stomach moves outward. Sip in a little more air when you think you've reached the

Don't Diss Yoga and Meditation

The benefits of yoga and meditation just got louder and clearer when a report in *Diabetes Research and Clinical Practice* discussed some startling findings from studies in India and Sweden. The studies showed that yoga and meditation, practiced for three months, reduced waist circumference, systolic blood pressure, and fasting blood sugar and triglyceride levels, and increased high-density lipoprotein (the good fats). In addition, at the end of the study periods, feelings of anxiety, stress, and depression were significantly decreased, and optimism was significantly increased. The researchers concluded that yoga not only helps in prevention of lifestyle diseases, but can also be a powerful adjunct therapy when diseases occur.

top of your lungs. Slowly exhale to a count of twenty, pushing every breath of air from your lungs. Continue for at least five rounds of deep breaths.

Get Balanced Fat on Your Brain

There's a reason why certain fats are necessary for survival and sanity. About two-thirds of our brains are composed of fat, and the protective sheath around communicating neurons is 70 percent fat. So in a sense we need fat to think and to maintain healthy brain function; in particular, the class of essential fatty acids called the omega-3s and omega-6s plays a crucial role in brain function as well as normal growth and development. This explains why foods such as salmon are often called "brain food." The omega-3 fats in salmon as well as other cold-water fish, avocados, walnuts, flaxseeds, and olives have numerous proven health benefits, including those that protect the heart. Healthy fats are at an all-time low in people's diets, whereas unhealthy fats (for example, saturated and trans), are at an all-time high. But it's the healthy fats that help fat-soluble vitamins such as A, D, E, and K move around the body, create sex hormones, build cell membranes, lower LDL (bad) cholesterol while raising HDL (good) cholesterol, and contribute to the health of skin, eyes, nails, and hair.

In the omega-6 family, gamma linoleic acid (also known as GLA) is one of the all-star anti-inflammatories and soothers. I mentioned GLA in chapter 5. Well known as a stress-reducing nutrient, GLA is largely deficient in the standard American diet because it's a rarer oil, found in seed oils such as borage oil, evening primrose oil, black currant oil, and hemp oil.

People are more likely to overdo other omega-6s from sources such as refined vegetable oils, which can *increase*—not decrease—inflammation. Soybean oil, for example, is ubiquitous in fast foods and processed foods; in fact, 20 percent of the calories in the American diet are estimated to come from this single source. This can create an imbalance of too many omega-6s and not enough omega-3s, which is partly being blamed for the rise of myriad diseases from asthma and heart disease to many forms of cancer and autoimmune diseases. The imbalance also may contribute to obesity, depression, dyslexia, and hyperactivity. One study showed that violence in a British prison dropped by 37 percent after omega-3 oils and vitamins were added to the prisoners' diets!

Getting a good balance of these fats is pretty easy. Simply reduce your consumption of processed and fast foods; also reduce the use and consumption of polyunsaturated vegetable oils (e.g., corn, sunflower, safflower, soy, and cottonseed). Switch to extra-virgin olive oil as much as possible (it's heart-stable, so use it to cook, too). Eat more oily fish (salmon, sardines, herring, mackerel, black cod, and bluefish) as well as walnuts, flaxseeds, and omega-3 fortified eggs. Don't forget to include a fish oil supplement in your daily vitamin regimen. All the recommendations made in chapters 4 and 5 will show you how to find the balance.

Get to Bed

While it sounds like a cliché, we do need "beauty sleep." Seemingly magical events happen when you're sleeping at night that just cannot happen during the day, and that help keep you healthy and, most of all, hydrated. Sleep medicine has come a long way in the past twenty years, and now it's a highly regarded field of study that continues to uncover alarming insights into the power of sleep in the support of health and longevity. Just about every system in the body is affected by the quality and amount of sleep you get at night. Sleep can dictate how much you eat, how fat you get, whether you can fight off infections, and how well you can cope with stress. The combined offenders of stress and sleep deprivation have been proven to steal precious water from cells. This helps to explain why "looking tired" typically means you're looking older and more dried out. Your skin's barrier function is compromised, and you're losing more water not only from your

What "Rested" Really Means

Fact: People who look well rested are foremost well hydrated. Sleep comes more easily to those who can retain healthy cellular water.

Are you well rested? This means not being able to fall asleep in a darkened room at midday. It's not normal to fall asleep if reading quietly in the afternoon or drift off at an afternoon meeting; sleep on airplanes in the daytime; feel drowsy after one glass of wine; sleep when you're a passenger in a car; fall asleep watching TV in the early evening; and need caffeine and open windows to drive two hours in the daytime.

skin cells but from every cell in your body. There's something to be said for looking "refreshed" upon waking from a good night's sleep or nap.

Sleep is not a state of inactivity. It's not as if our bodies press PAUSE for a few hours during the dark. Much to the contrary, a lot goes on during sleep at the cellular level to ensure that we can live another day. Clearly, a night of poor sleep or no sleep at all won't kill you, but prolonged sleep deprivation can have unintended consequences, not to mention put you at high risk for an accident.

Personal experience alone tells you what sleeplessness can do: make you look haggard, moody, depressed, and downright negative about things in life. It also can encourage you to overeat, drink too much caffeine, scream at your spouse and kids, and dodge workouts and sex because you're just too tired. Proof of sleep's profound role in our lives also has been proven over and over again in laboratory and clinical studies. Among the many side effects of poor sleep habits are hypertension, confusion, memory loss, the inability to learn new things, weight gain, obesity, cardiovascular disease, and depression. How are these things possible?

First, it helps to understand that sleep commands much of our well-being through our biological clocks—and I'm not referring to the one women talk about with regard to their fertility. Every one of us has a so-called circadian rhythm, a natural cycle of biological activity that changes throughout the twenty-four-hour day. This rhythm revolves around our sleep habits or, more specifically, the shifts from daytime to nighttime. A healthy day/night cycle is tethered to our normal hormonal secretion patterns, from those associated with our eating patterns to those that relate to stress, metabolism, and cellular recovery and renewal. The stress hormone cortisol, for example, should be highest in the morning and progressively decrease as the day wears on. It should be at its nadir after 11:00 P.M., at which point melatonin levels peak. This is the hormone that tells you it's time to sleep (and probably starts to get pumped out of your pineal gland at about 9:00 P.M., when the body senses it's dark outside). Once released, melatonin slows body function and lowers blood pressure and, in turn, core body temperature, so you're prepared to sleep. Higher melatonin levels will allow for more deep sleep, which helps maintain healthy levels of growth hormone, thyroid hormone, and male and female sex hormones. If you've ever had a tough time winding down at night due to stress, you may be secreting too much cortisol, which competes with the sleep-enhancing melatonin.

Lots of hormones are associated with sleep, some of which rely on sleep to get released. As soon as you hit deep sleep, about twenty to thirty minutes after you first close your eyes, and then a couple more times throughout the night in your sleep cycle, your pituitary gland at the base of your brain releases high levels of growth hormone (GH)—the most it's going to secrete in twenty-four hours. Growth hormone does more than just stimulate growth and cell reproduction; it also refreshes cells and restores skin's elasticity, as well as enhances the movement of amino acids through cell membranes. Growth hormone aids in your ability to maintain an ideal weight, too, effectively telling your cells to back off on

The Hormone That Keeps on Giving

Growth hormone affects almost every cell in the body, renewing the skin and bones; regenerating the heart, liver, lungs, and kidneys; and bringing back organ and tissue function to more youthful levels. Growth hormone also revitalizes the immune system, lowers the risk factors of heart attack and stroke, improves oxygen uptake, and even helps prevent osteoporosis.

using carbs for energy and use fat instead. Without adequate sleep, GH stays locked up in the pituitary, which negatively affects your proportions of fat to muscle. Over time, low GH levels are associated with high fat and low lean muscle.

I see lots of patients who complain of weight gain but don't think twice about their sleep habits as they rethink their diet and exercise regimens. Yet the two digestive hormones tied to sleep habits actually control your feelings of hunger and appetite. Ghrelin (your "go eat" hormone) gets secreted by the stomach when it's empty and sends a message to your brain that you need to eat. When your stomach is full, fat cells send out the other hormone—leptin—so your brain gets the message that you can stop eating now. One of the most exciting findings revealed in the past decade has been showing how out of whack these hormones get after insufficient sleep. When people are allowed just four hours of sleep a night for two nights, they experience a 20 percent drop in leptin and an increase in ghrelin. They also have a marked increase (about 24 percent) in hunger and appetite. And what do they gravitate toward? Calorie-dense, high-carbohydrate foods such as sweets, salty snacks, and starchy foods. Sleep loss essentially deceives your body into believing it's hungry when it's not, and it also tricks you into craving foods that can sabotage a healthy diet. What's more, because we need sleep to metabolize glucose properly, sleep loss over time can lead to diabetes.

Sleep Keeps You Smart

No joke, it's been proven that sleep inspires insight. By restructuring new memory representations, sleep facilitates the extraction of explicit knowledge and insightful behavior. Put simply, sleep keeps you sharp, quick-witted, creative, and able to process information in an instant. Losing as few as one and a half hours for just one night reduces daytime alertness by about a third.

Sleep deprivation impairs the body's ability to use insulin, the hormone responsible for keeping stable blood sugar levels.

I can go on and on about the value of sleep and the casualties of not getting enough. Most of us don't get the sleep we need. Sleep deprivation is epidemic. On average, we get an hour less sleep per day than we did forty years ago, and roughly two thirds of us complain that sleep deprivation cuts into our life and well-being. In fact, sleep may have a greater influence on your ability to enjoy your day than household income and even marital status. One study found that an extra hour of sleep had more of an impact on how a group of women felt throughout the day than earning more money a year.

Everyone has a different sleep need. The "eight hour" rule is general, but not necessarily the ideal number for you. Most people need seven to nine hours, and chances are you know what your number is. If you feel like a drag after a six-hour night, then clearly you need to aim for more sleep. Think of the last time you went on vacation and slept like a baby for more hours a night than usual. *That* is probably your perfect number. Poor sleep catches up to most people, and it's not physically possible to make up a sleep loss. Despite what many people attempt to do, shifting your sleep habits on the weekends to "catch up" can sabotage a healthy circadian rhythm.

Stress and hormonal aging are the two big culprits to poor sleep, which is why it's important to establish what's called

Top Ten To-Dos

1. Have a good day, daily.
2. Eat an extra egg once a week.
3. Deep-breathe daily.
4. Take a relaxing bath with candles or have a massage, once a week.
5. Stand up straight daily.
6. Take a new path once a week.
7. Give/get a bear hug daily.
8. Splurge on your appearance once a month.
9. Lie in bed an extra ten minutes once a week.
10. Take a wellness day once a month.

healthy "sleep hygiene"—the habits that make for a restful night's sleep regardless of factors such as age, stress, and underlying medical conditions that can disrupt sleep. The goal is to minimize those factors' effects on us so we can welcome peaceful sleep.

Eight Tips to Sound Sleep

1. Go to bed and wake up at the same time seven days a week, weekends included. Try not to fall into a cycle of burning the midnight oil on Saturday night and then sleeping until noon on Sunday. Stick to the same schedule. Your body and energy levels will love it.
2. Set aside at least thirty minutes before bedtime to unwind and prepare for sleep. Avoid stimulating activities (e.g., work, cleaning, being on the computer, watching TV dramas that get your adrenaline running). Try soaking in a warm bath or engaging in some light stretching. Once you're in bed, do some light reading and push any anxieties aside.

3. Don't let your to-do list or worries take control. Early in the evening—say, right after dinner—write out tasks you have yet to complete that week (not tonight!) and prioritize them realistically. Add any particular worries you might have. If these notes begin to talk to you when you're trying to go to sleep, tell yourself *It's time to focus on sleep. Everything will be okay. You're tired and will have a productive day tomorrow. You're relaxed and at peace. The body needs to sleep and is ready for it*.
4. Reserve the bedroom for sleep only. Remove distracting electronics and gadgets and keep it clean, cool, and dark.
5. Avoid caffeine after 2:00 P.M. and avoid exercise at least three hours before bedtime. Watch alcohol intake at dinner. Keep in mind that heavy foods too close to bedtime can be a digestive distraction. (Skip another helping of Mom's meat loaf as a bedtime snack and have a piece of toast with a spread of natural peanut butter.)
6. Look for GABA (gamma-aminobutyric acid) for your nighttime facial products or supplements. This helps your muscles to relax so they can repair themselves

Aromatherapy Is Real

A great deal of scientific literature suggests that certain scents can influence mood, anxiety, immune function, and even skin health. Add some aromatherapy to your bath, or keep an essential (natural) oil by your bedside. Lavender, for example, has known sleep-enhancing qualities. Other aromas linked to sensations of relaxation include rose, vanilla, and lemongrass. You can find sleep-friendly oils to dab under your nose for a calming effect. Once an essential oil is inhaled, nerves at the top of your nose carry it to the part of the brain that controls heart rate, memory, and hormone balance, among other things.

maximally during this important rejuvenating period. You also may want to take some extra antioxidants and hydrating agents at nighttime. Flooding the body with more nutrients will fuel your cellular repair shop that opens during sleep.

7. Try valerian herbal tea or a chamomile blend before bedtime. Keep a sachet of lavender by your bed and take a whiff before hitting the pillow. Lavender has known sleep-inducing effects.
8. Take a d-e-e-p breath and release. On your back with your eyes closed and your body stretched out, hands by your side, palms facing up, begin to squeeze and release your muscles, starting with your head and face and working down to your toes. Breathe in deeply and slowly, telling yourself *I will fall asleep. I am going to sleep*.

At my company, we've formulated a supplement to encourage the onset of sleep by incorporating GABA plus a low dose of melatonin, the hormone your body begins to pump into your bloodstream when night falls. Melatonin readies your body for sleep, and since our bodies produce less melatonin over time, some people find that occasional use of a small boost, through supplementation, can ease them back into a normal sleep cycle, even though it is highly unlikely that they have a serious melatonin deficiency. In all likelihood, establishing better bedtime habits can be the biggest part of the solution.

The Whole Story

The idea that the body is a whole unit and that no single piece of it—an organ, an area of skin, a heartbeat, a strand of hair—can be understood without considering every other piece to the body cannot be understated. I have firsthand experience as to how the body requires a three-pronged perspective.

Last year, I suffered torn cartilage in one of my knees, and like most people I initially assumed that I had twisted it during exercise or my daily movements. I kept focusing on the knee and searching for the solution to fixing the problem and alleviating my pain quickly. Suffice it to say I had my traditional medical doctor's hat on as I went about the typical troubleshooting. I had an important lesson to learn, though. And it would further affirm every belief I had in my theory about aging and the workings of the human body.

I confess that I wasn't able to help myself when it came to my knee. When I started physical therapy, my therapist asked me to perform a simple task: walk across the room. She then smiled like she knew something I didn't. "Your right leg is shorter than the other," she told me. I looked down in disbelief, wondering how I could have missed this important fact about my body this long. But it was true. My asymmetrical legs had led me to unwittingly overcorrect this disparity by pulling up on my right leg and thus weakening my left leg, to the point when it began to manifest itself in the knee. The solution wasn't about the knee at all. It was about correcting my imbalanced walk. With the help of orthotics in my shoes to give my right side a lift, I was cured. My lower back thanked me, too.

Whether you're suffering from a specific pain in your body, or just the pain of too much stress, I encourage you to begin to think more globally about your body. Throughout this book I've underscored the importance of realizing the interconnectedness of the whole body, and I'll say it again: as you treat your whole body well and infuse it with what it needs to reduce damage to its cells, you'll reduce your body's stress load—the load that causes you to age and become afflicted with disease. Regardless of what people tell you about how to age, if your cells are damaged, wherever they are, they cannot function at their highest level. The promise of the Water Secret is to show you how to ensure the highest level of functioning of every cell in your body.

How are your cells today? Do they carry the burden of an unhealthy lifestyle? Is the stress in your life choking their livelihood? Will they be there for you when you need them to function at 110 percent to prevent disease and be your sentinels of health? If you could get a score on your cellular health, what do you think that would be? What would be your Murad number?

At my Inclusive Health Spa in Los Angeles, my team and I are currently pioneering a new method of evaluating health based on the Water Secret. Every day we learn new knowledge about the body and what it means to be healthy. I trust we will only continue to learn more as newer studies bear out the mysteries of life and of aging.

EPILOGUE

Your Best Is Yet to Come

Ignore the naysayers from without and, more importantly, those from within. Allow yourself to achieve your maximum potential.

By now I hope you've gained not only a lot of information on ways to improve your quality of life and health, but also a greater appreciation for your body's inherent healing capacity when it's bathed in nutrients and well hydrated at the cellular level. I applaud you for your decision to take better care of yourself, no matter how small a step you take starting today. Just picking up this book moves you ahead! And as you no doubt understand, through personal experience alone, the way you look and feel says so much about you—your confidence, your courage and character, and even your faith in yourself and the world at large.

Our knowledge about aging and disease, and the consequences to the choices we make regarding our lifestyles, will only continue to expand. I'm certain that what we will discover in the future will reinforce the necessity of honoring the Water Secret and its techniques for maintaining better lifestyles that can support our longevity. Remember, we want to live healthfully for as long as possible. We live in a youth-obsessed culture that sadly idolizes the young and casts aside the old, but the quest to "look young" does not have to be about vanity at all. There's nothing wrong with looking as youthful as you can regardless of your chronological age. The word *youthful* is synonymous with healthful. When you're healthy, you look and feel young, and there's absolutely nothing wrong with that.

We live in an exciting time in health, medicine, and wellness—characterized by increasingly more access to better lifestyle habits. Farmer's markets are the norm in many parts of the United States. Medical spas are cropping up to bridge that tremendous gap between traditional medicine and attention to the details of emotion, relaxation, and holistic medicine. Every day we hear about breakthroughs in pharmaceuticals and learn about new drugs that can help us treat or prevent a wide variety of diseases. We also have countless resources to help us make the changes we know we need to make. Yet, ironically, our struggle with certain health problems has never been greater. We still have high rates of heart disease, cancer, diabetes, obesity, sleep apnea, and depression, to name a few. My hope is that the Water Secret helps you to put all this overwhelming information into perspective and adopt a new approach to wellness that can capitalize on all these great advancements in health.

As a physician, I see patients every day who have a variety of issues caused by their poor diet and fitness, their general failure to simply take better emotional care, and their failure to pay as much attention to skin health as they do to their internal health.

And while I do see patients who have a clean bill of health with the exception of a dermatological issue, I also see people who are battling a life-threatening illness such as cancer. In fact, one of my patients in the past year was a woman fighting a tough war on a particularly invasive type of lung cancer. Suzanne's visits with me coincided with one of the most difficult periods in her life as she underwent chemotherapy and radiation and tried to put her life into perspective. She also endured invasive surgical procedures in combating the cancer.

I admired Suzanne's strength and tenacity, but I also sensed that she was depressed because of the cancer and what that meant for her future. I told her to stop thinking about the cancer as a fatal illness and instead start thinking of it as a chronic illness such as diabetes. That became a turning point for her, giving her hope and a new perspective that could focus on life rather than death.

Despite all the medical treatments Suzanne underwent for her cancer, she kept up with the protocol I had given her to address her Inclusive Health. Unwilling to give up her daily regimen of tending to her skin and paying attention to her diet and stress levels, Suzanne expressed to me numerous times that had she not maintained her self-care, she would not have felt so good as she endured all those cancer treatments. In fact, she credited her nutrition and supplements as the reason why she felt more energetic and relatively healthy following chemotherapy versus previous times, when she wasn't as careful about nutrition and supplementing. This didn't surprise me. When you give your body what it needs to work optimally, you give your body what it needs to heal itself as best it can and leave you feeling as good as possible. Just because you have cancer or any other illness doesn't mean you give up on the rest of you.

This is an important point. Remember, the Water Secret and the notion of Inclusive Health are universal—not just about making healthy people healthier or curing a specific illness. It's not just about preventive medicine or treatment, either. Inclusive Health is about looking at the body as a whole in a three-pronged manner so you can be the best you can be at any age and under any circumstance or condition. All too often we think of medicine as treating disease, or we see preventive medicine as staving off a particular illness such as cancer or heart disease. This is not the express goal of Inclusive Health. The goal, rather, is much larger and more comprehensive: to use the science of the Water Secret to renew the body and all its component parts through an approach that begins and ends with health on the cellular level.

Let me give you another example from my own experience. During the writing of this book, I had already been living by the Water Secret for years. I felt at the top of my health game and in pretty good shape. But then something happened unexpectedly: I suffered a detached retina in my right eye, which made me housebound for a few weeks as I let the eye heal. This also meant avoiding a lot of my normal activities. What was I going to do?

It turns out that my recuperation became an opportunity to tap a hidden talent. The previous year, during a stay in Ojai, California, I took a one-hour art class for fun. Without much direction, I picked up the paintbrush and started painting. My instructor, pleased by what I had done on the canvas, suggested I keep working on this talent and get a good set of art supplies. I remember her telling me, "I don't want you to be spoiled by someone directing you." Clearly, she wanted me to have fun and find time to experiment with this skill on a regularly.

Flash forward about a year. Here I was cooped up at home with a bad eye, and that set of art supplies that I had purchased long ago had never been used. So I fished out the supplies from a closet, sat at my desk, and started to paint. And paint some more. And some more. The dozens of pieces I've since created now adorn my office. They are constant reminders of this other talent I have that's gone unnoticed for most of my life. They also remind me to stop my typical routine and just play with my creativity once in a while. I sometimes wonder what else I will discover about myself. Out of a painful and frustrating experience with the eye came this wonderful revelation about myself. I've always said that the best is yet to come, and I firmly believe that. Not just for me, but for everyone who puts a positive effort and attitude forward and reveres the tenets of Inclusive Health no matter what's going on in his or her life.

Your dedication to nurturing your body and skin from the inside out will reward you in so many fantastic ways—not just today, but every day forward for the rest of your life. I wish you the best of luck in your journey, and I encourage you to come back to this book when you need reminders about healthy living. I can't think of a more rewarding life than being able to help people look younger, feel healthier, and live happier. And remember to visit me at www.thewatersecretbook.com

for continued support. As I stated earlier, I can't think of a more rewarding life than being able to help people look younger, feel healthier, and live happier. Remember, your best is yet to come; you just have to allow it to enter. I leave you with this thought:

Each of us is born with a unique commodity called life. It is stressed by the environment, and it is up to us to make the best of it.

Your partner in health,
Howard Murad, M.D.

Acknowledgments

This book reflects the culmination of not just my lifetime work in the health care and wellness industry, but also my collaboration with a small village of bright, passionate people who surround me every day. An entire book could be filled with the names of those who have shaped who I am today, for I owe everyone I've ever worked with and treated through the years a heartfelt thank-you. The unwavering support of family members, friends, and colleagues also have paved the path to this book. Your guidance, insights, and feedback have been indispensable; *The Water Secret* is as much yours as it is mine.

First, I give a resounding thanks to my patients, who teach me daily about how the body works. Their stories and experiences are what challenge me to constantly seek fresh perspectives on what makes us sick and why we age, so I can then address their needs and help them to optimize their vitality. The Water Secret as the driving force of my message wouldn't exist without them.

I am eternally grateful to my wife and best friend, Loralee, whose daily encouragement, good humor, and wisdom keep me inspired and focused. And to my children, Hilarie, Jeff, and Elizabeth, who are always there for me when I need advice and have been gracious champions of my career and dedication to health. Richard, I thank you for playing such a big part in my life and career.

When I first had lunch with Jill Marsal about doing a book, I knew it was finally time to share the knowledge that I had been collecting through years of research, much of which could be used to enhance the health of millions. Jill quickly saw the passion in me and embraced my philosophy. Thank you, Jill, for enabling me to finally reach those people; your leadership and steadfast commitment to this project from its very early stages have been invaluable.

Thank you Kristin Loberg, my writing partner, who listened to my many scientific talks, accompanied me on days I treated patients, digested copious medical research I shared with her from around the world, heard numerous stories about the Water Secret improving the health of my patients, and transformed it all into an engaging, simple piece of writing. Keeping the layman's ear in mind, she skillfully helped me craft a compelling and convincing message about the role cellular water plays in our health and how you can take charge of your life and looks in ways you never thought possible.

To the entire team at Murad, Inc., and the Murad Medical Group, whose loyal support elevates me and makes my job easy and the delivery of my message to the world possible. Thanks especially to Tracey Sameyah, Lori Jacobus, Paula Coyne, and Julieta Vidal-Lubin. Thanks also to Harris Shepard for handling my PR all these years so thoughtfully and creatively, and to David Ratner and Shirley Sandler at Newman Communications.

To Paul Williams and Monica Schuloff Smith, my trusted duo for facilitating my scientific papers and their submission for publication.

To my publishing stewards at John Wiley & Sons, especially Christel Winkler, John Simko, Aaditi Shah, and Matthew Smollon. Your enthusiasm and ideas have made for a sharper piece of work and a stronger marketing campaign.

Many thanks to my dear friends who help me celebrate life and live up to the Water Secret. Thanks especially to Dr. Bill Shellow for your continuous support and my tireless hiking comrade Dr. David Stern.

To my grandchildren, Lilly, Devyn, Reese, and Travis, whom I learn from every day and who keep me feeling young. And to everyone else in the Murad family camp—you know who you are and each of you has been pivotal more than you know. Thank you for making my life that much richer and accomplished.

I'm known for saying that I chose good parents, and though they are no longer living, a special thanks goes out to Albert and Rachel Murad for nurturing me into a thoughtful, productive adult who keeps trying to make the world a better—healthier—place.

Index

abdominal fat, 167
acidic foods, 142–144
acne, 43–44, 133–135, 185–186, 195, 228
acute stress, 219
adrenaline, 225
adrenocorticotropic hormone (ACTH), 225
aerobic exercise, 171–172. *See also* exercise
aging process, 37–40
  hormone replacement therapy (HRT) and, 48–50
  reversing, 16–21, 46–48, 55–56
  three-pronged approach to, 50–55
  types of aging, 41–45
  from wastewater, 40–41
air toxins, 80–86
alcohol, 155, 167
almonds, 114
alpha-hydroxy acid (AHA), 8, 38, 187–188
alpha-linoleic acid (ALA), 149
amino acids, 40, 51–52, 138, 199–201
analgesics, 61
androgens, 229
andropause, 43
animal-based foods, 65, 72, 142. *See also individual names of foods and recipes*
antioxidants, 59, 66, 138, 146–147, 152–153, 189–193
apples, 200
apricots, 62, 67
aromatherapy, 244
Asian diet, 65, 67–68
Asian Stir-Fry Vegetables with Skinless Chicken or Tofu, 125–127
aspartame, 142
avocados, 110

bacteria, 84
Balsamic Vinaigrette Dressing, 123
basal metabolic rate, 169
beans, 64–65
berries, 66, 146. *See also* goji berries
beta-carotene, 67
beta-endorphins, 228
beverages, 104, 155–156, 167. *See also* recipes
bicep curls, 172
Biological Value Scale, 145–146
blood vessels, 52, 167
"blue zones," 215
body composition analysis, 163, 166
body fat, 71–73, 162, 165–168, 169
bone health, 171–172
Botox, 184

Bragg's Liquid Aminos, 105
brain health, 237
bran, 111–112
breakfast, 155–157, 235. *See also* meal plans
breathing exercises, 100, 235–236, 245
broccoli, 105
brown fat, 166
B vitamins, 150–151, 153

caffeine, 95, 198
calcium, 72, 154–155
calories, 65, 156, 169, 174
cancer, 37, 141–144, 252–253
capsaicin, 77–78
carbohydrates (carbs), 107
carotenoids, 67
Carroll, Aaron E., 64
carrots, 64
catechins, 190
celebration, 101
cells
  aging process and, 39, 54
  cellular water, 3–4, 15–16, 18–21, 25, 168
  deterioration of, 62–63
  membrane of, 25
Cellular Water Secret Smoothie
  about, 102–103
  recipe, 119
cellulite, 199
ceramides, 194
cheese, 64
chicken, 64
  Chicken and Black Bean Burrito, 127
  Chicken Vegetable Soup, 120–121
children, 223–224
chili peppers, 77–78
cholesterol, 145
chromosomes, 16, 27
chronic stress, 219–220
citrus, 116, 146
cleansers, 187–188, 197–198, 202, 204
coenzyme Q10, 190
collagen, 40–41, 43, 51–52
  in moisturizers, 194
  from nutrition, 141
  plant-based foods and, 60
  for wrinkles, 184–185, 196
community involvement, 97–98
connectedness, 229, 232–233
connective tissue, 40, 51, 62
corticotropin-releasing hormone (CRH), 225
cortisol, 226, 231
cosmeceutical ingredients, 187
Cultural Stress, 5, 210, 213–217, 245–247
  antidotes to, 230–245 (*See also* relaxation)
  connectedness and, 229, 232–233
  defined, 220–222
  effect on health, 228–230
  emotions and, 225, 226–228
  inflammation and, 223
  isolation and, 97–98, 222–223
  science of stress and, 217–220
  stress attacks and, 225–226
  stress in children and, 223–224
  technology and, 222, 233–234
  traffic and, 224
  work and, 221
curcumin, 76–77
cytoplasm, 40

dairy, 142
deep-breathing exercises, 100, 235–236, 245
delayed onset muscle soreness (DOMS), 172–173
depression, 222
dermatologists, 204
detoxification (detox), 82, 188–189
dietary fat, 70, 147–150, 237
digestion, 71, 84, 152, 174–175
dihydrotestosterone (DHT), 205
dinner. *See* meal plans
Dinner Party Secret Salad, 124
DNA, 56
docosahexaenoic acid (DHA), 149–150
Dr. Brand, 7–8
dry skin, 206
dry skin brushing, 188–189
durian, 147, 201

eggplant, 64
eggs, 17, 145–146
elastin, 40–41, 43, 51–52, 60, 141
ellagic acid, 66
emotional health, 95–96
  aging process and, 55
  Cultural Stress and, 215–216, 225, 226–228
  depression and, 222
  exercise and, 176
  food-mood connection, 139
endosperm, 111–112
environmental aging, 42
episodic acute stress, 219
essential fatty acids (EFAs), 66, 91, 110, 138, 147–149, 153, 237–238
estrogen, 43–44, 145–146
ethnobotany, 59–61
exercise, 19, 91–92
  bone health and, 171–172
  finding time for, 176–177
  hydration and, 161–164, 177–178
  maintaining exercise routine, 164–165
  measuring progress from, 175–176
  metabolism and, 168–171
  mood and, 176
  muscle soreness and, 172–174
  posture and, 174–175
  for relaxation, 231
  types of body fat and, 165–168
exfoliators, 187–188, 197–198, 204
extra-virgin olive oil, 107, 149
eyes, 198

face-lifts, 184
facials, 204
fat. *See* body fat; dietary fat; essential fatty acids (EFAs)
fiber, 71–73, 84
fish, 64, 83, 148–149
Flax-Goji Golden Citrus Dressing
  about, 113
  recipe, 122
flaxseeds, 114
food
  acidic, 142–144
  animal-based, 65, 72, 142
  food-mood connection, 139
  labels, 73
  as medicine, 61–62
  organic, 136, 150–151
  preparation of, 65, 84, 108–109
  processed foods, 70, 72–73
  storage, 149
  See also recipes; *individual names of foods*
food pyramid (U.S. Department of Agriculture), 138
free radicals, 23, 189, 190, 192
fruits
  low acid-forming foods, 143
  organic, 151
  recommended, 74
  structured water from, 140
  variety of, 115
  See also plant-based foods; recipes; *individual names of fruits*

gamma-aminobutyric acid (GABA), 244
gamma-linoleic acid (GLA), 149–150, 237–238
garlic, 78
germ (from grains), 111–112
ghrelin, 241
ginger, 75–76
ginkgo biloba, 190
glucosamine, 51, 91, 152
glycolic peel, 188
glycosaminoglycans (GAGs), 51
goji berries
  about, 68, 146–147
  Flax-Goji Golden Citrus Dressing, 113
grains, 64, 105, 107, 111–112, 140–141. *See also* recipes
green tea, 190
growth hormone (GH), 240–241

habits, changing, 99
hair loss, 204–205
happiness, 231–232
health. *See* wellness
heart attack, 224
hobbies, 96, 231–232
homemade scrub and detox bath, 189

homeostasis, 51
hormonal aging, 42–45, 145, 242–243
hormone replacement therapy (HRT), 48–50
humectants, 194
Hummus, 129
hyaluronic acid, 172–174, 184–185, 194
hydration
  aging process and, 50
  from exercise, 161–164, 177–178
  health and, 21–23
  myths about drinking water and, 63–64
  from nutrient-dense food sources, 141
  from plant-based foods, 62–65, 70–71, 74–75
  plant-based foods and, 90
  structured water from fruits and vegetables, 140
  supplements and, 90–91
  wastewater and, 22, 40–41
  water in skin, 183
  wellness water, 22–23
  See also plant-based foods
hydrators, 194
hydroquinone, 197
hydroxy acids, 189–193
hyperpigmentation, 196–197
hypothalamic-pituitary-adrenal (HPA) axis, 225, 227

immunity, 182–183
Inclusive Health care
  defined, 5–9
  integrative and preventive medicine *vs.*, 26–28
  as universal, 253
  See also wellness
inflammation, 23–24, 60, 223
insulin, 170, 242
integrative health, 26–28
intrinsic aging, 42
iron, 72
isolation, 97–98, 222–223

jam/spreads, 106–107
jobs, 96, 221
joint fluids, 172–174
journals, 93–94

kale, 117
Kavli crispbread, 102
kidneys, 70–71, 81–82

labels, 73
lactic acid, 116, 173
lean tissue, 162
lecithin, 40, 91, 138, 144–145, 153
leptin, 241
licorice, 200, 201
lifestyle, 89–90
  aging process and, 37
  celebration and, 101
  eating plant-based foods and, 69
  emotional health and, 95–96
  exercise and, 91–92
  hydrating with plant-based foods and, 90
  hydrating with supplements and, 90–91
  relaxation and, 98–100
  self-discovery and, 92–94
  skin care routine and, 98
  sleep and, 94–95
  volunteering and, 97–98
  See also meal plans
lipids, 40
Li Qing Uyen, 68
liver, 81–82
lunch. *See* meal plans

makeup removal, 203
massage therapy, 234–235
meal plans, 101–102
  beverages, 102
  Days 1 through 10, 102–117
  improvement in health from, 118
  recipes for, 119–130
meat, 142
medical-spa industry, 210
medicine, 47, 61–62, 95
meditation, 100, 236
melatonin, 228, 240, 245
memory, 242

men
  alcohol consumption by, 167
  andropause and, 43
  skin care for, 207–208
menopause, 42–45, 49, 197–198
metabolism, 168–171
microdermabrasion treatment, 188
microwaving, 108
minerals
  absorption of, 72
  supplements, 152
moisturizers, 203
  effective ingredients in, 191
  uses for, 193–194
Monterey Bay Aquarium Seafood Watch, 83
multimorbidity, 47
multivitamins, 91, 152
Murad, Howard, 7–12, 199, 254
Murad Inclusive Health Spa, 8–9, 69, 164
Murad Skin Research Laboratory, 7
muscle
  pain, 157–158
  strength training and, 170–171
  weight and, 162
mushrooms, 200
mustard seed, 79

neuro-immuno-cutaneous-endocrine (NICE) network, 183, 227
nucleus, 40
nutrients, 133–135
  aging process and, 51–52
  antioxidants and, 146–147
  beverages and, 155–156
  breakfast and, 155–157
  B vitamins and, 150–151
  cancer cells and foods, 141–144
  eggs and, 145–146
  essential ingredients for, 138
  fats and, 147–150
  lecithin and, 144–145
  pain relief and, 157–158
  Pitcher of Health for, 136–137, 138–140
  relaxation and, 235
  sleep and, 241
  stevia and, 151
  supplements, 151–155
  water from nutrient-dense food sources, 141
  whole grains and, 140–141
  See also minerals; recipes; vitamins; *individual names of foods*
nuts, 66–67, 114

oatmeal, 105
oily skin, 206
olive oil
  about, 107, 149
  Olive Oil and Lemon Juice Dressing, 122–123
  Olive Oil and Red Wine Vinegar Dressing, 123
omega-3 fatty acids, 91, 114, 237
omega-6 fatty acids, 237
oranges, 62, 116
organelles, 54–55
organic products, 83, 136, 150–151
osteoporosis, 171–172
outdoor recreation, 99
oxidation, 189

pain, 157–158, 172–174
parasympathetic nervous system, 236
pasta, 64
peaches, 64
peptides, 199–201
pesticides, 74–75
Phase Angle (PA), 15–16
  exercise and, 165–166
  self-assessment of wellness and, 32
  test for, 19
phloretin, 200
phosphatidylcholine, 138
phytochemicals, 66–67, 83
Pilates, 175
pistachios, 67
Pitcher of Health, 110, 111, 116, 136–137, 138–140
plant-based foods, 59–61, 90
  air toxins and, 80–86
  Asian diet and, 65, 67–68

plant-based foods (*continued*)
- detoxification and, 82
- fiber from, 71–73, 84
- food as medicine, 61–62
- hydration from, 62–65, 70–71
- importance of, 65–66
- making dietary changes and, 86
- phytochemicals in, 66–67, 83
- recommended fruits and vegetables, 74–75
- shopping for, 68–70
- spices and health benefits, 75–80

pollutants, 80–86
polyphenols, 66–67
pomegranates, 59, 62, 66, 200–201
pore size, 206
positive-note journals, 94
posture, 174–175
prebiotics, 84
preventive medicine, 26–28
protein, 110, 116
puberty, 184–185

raw vegetables, 65, 108, 115
recipes
- Asian Stir-Fry Vegetables with Skinless Chicken or Tofu, 125–127
- Balsamic Vinaigrette Dressing, 123
- Cellular Water Secret Smoothie, 119
- Chicken and Black Bean Burrito, 127
- Chicken Vegetable Soup, 120–121
- Dinner Party Secret Salad, 124
- Flax-Goji Golden Citrus Dressing, 122
- Hummus, 129
- Olive Oil and Lemon Juice Dressing, 122–123
- Olive Oil and Red Wine Vinegar Dressing, 123
- Roasted Greens, 129–130
- Steamed Tofu, 127
- Steamed Vegetables with Marinara Sauce, 125
- Sumptuous Veggie Scramble, 120
- Tasty Turkey Scramble, 156
- Tomato Salsa, 128
- Tropical Protein Smoothie, 119
- Vegetarian Chili, 128
- Vegetarian Split Pea with Barley Soup, 121–122
- Veggie Antioxidant Juice Smoothie, 119–120
- Veggie Sandwich on Whole-Wheat Pita, 124–125
- Water Secret Crunchie Smoothie, The, 156

relaxation, 98–100, 230–231
- aromatherapy for, 244
- brain health and dietary fat, 237–238
- breaking routine for, 235
- connectedness and, 232–233
- deep-breathing exercises, 100, 235–236, 245
- exercise for, 231
- hobbies for, 231–232
- meditation for, 236
- nutrition and, 235
- sleep and rest for, 238–244
- technology and, 233–234
- touch therapy for, 234–235
- yoga for, 236
- *See also* Cultural Stress

rest, 238–244
resting metabolism, 168–171
retinoids, 67, 195
retinols, 196
Roasted Greens, 129–130
rosacea, 228

salads
- about, 116
- Dinner Party Secret Salad, 124

salmon, 64
salt, 70–71, 75
Seafood Watch (Monterey Bay Aquarium), 83
self-discovery, 92–94
Selye, Hans, 218
serotonin, 228
shampoos, 205
skin, thickness of, 207
skin care, 8–9, 181–182
- aggressive approaches to, 184–185, 188, 209–210
- aging process and, 42–45, 53–55

alpha-hydroxy acids for, 187–188
developing routine for, 98
for different age groups, 185–186
dry skin brushing for, 188–189
hair loss and, 204–205
homemade scrub and detox bath, 189
immunity and, 182–183
for men, 207–208
moisturizers for, 191, 193–194
nutrition and, 133–135, 141, 146 (*See also* nutrients)
peptides and, 199–201
personalized regimen for, 201–204
products and treatments for, 184–185
professional help for, 204
skin types and, 205–206
special ingredients for special situations, 195–199
topical antioxidants for, 189–193
vitamin D and, 183, 208–209
skins, of fruits/vegetables, 73
skin types, 205–206
sleep, 94–95, 238–244
snacks. *See* meal plans
soy lecithin granules, 144
spices, 75–80
spine, 175
Steamed Tofu, 127
Steamed Vegetables with Marinara Sauce, 125
stevia, 151
stir frying
about, 109
Asian Stir-Fry Vegetables with Skinless Chicken or Tofu, 125–127
stratum corneum, 55
strength training, 170–171. *See also* exercise; muscle
stress
defined, 217–218
types of, 218–222
See also Cultural Stress
stretch marks, 198
sugar, 70, 142
sugar substitutes, 142, 151
sumac, 78–79
Sumptuous Veggie Scramble, 120
sunscreen, 189, 192, 196, 206
supplements, 90–91, 151–155, 157–158
sympathetic nervous system, 236
Szent-Gyorgi von Nagyrapolt, Albert, 16–17

Tasty Turkey Scramble, 156
technology, 222, 233–234
teenagers, 185–186
telomeres, 16, 27
testosterone, 43, 169
thirst, 64
thirties, skin care during, 186
tomatoes
about, 64
Tomato Salsa, 128
toner, 202–203
topical antioxidants, 38, 189–193
tortillas, 64
Touch Research Institute, 234
touch therapy, 234–235
toxins, 80–86, 188–189
traffic, 221, 224
Tropical Protein Smoothie, 119
turmeric, 76–77
twenties, skin care during, 186
Twiggy-Fat Syndrome, 166

ultraviolet (UV) rays, 183, 193, 208–209
University of Inclusive Health, 9
U.S. Department of Agriculture, 138

valerian herbal tea, 245
vegetable juice drinks, 104
vegetables
green, leafy, 117
list of recommended vegetables, 74–75
low acid-forming foods, 143
organic, 151
salads, 116
structured water from, 140
See also plant-based foods; recipes; *individual names of vegetables*
Vegetarian Chili, 128
Vegetarian Split Pea with Barley Soup, 121–122

Veggie Antioxidant Juice Smoothie, 119–120
Veggie Sandwich on Whole-Wheat Pita, 124–125
visceral fat, 166–168
vitamins
  A, 67, 152, 189, 195
  B, 150–151, 153
  brain health and, 237
  C, 38, 62, 146, 189, 191–192
  D, 183, 208–209
  E, 152, 189
  multivitamins, 91, 152
  topical, 189
volunteering, 97–98
Vreeman, Rachel C., 6

walnuts, 66–67, 114
wastewater, 22, 40–41
watermelon, 64
"water retention," 18, 26
Water Secret, 251–255
  cell hydration and, 3–4, 15–16, 18–21
  diet additions and, 4
  goal of, 49
  Inclusive Health care and, 5–9
  plant-based foods and hydration, 63
  reversing aging process and, 46–48
  "water retention" *vs.*, 26
Water Secret Crunchie Smoothie, The, 156
weight
  exercise and body fat, 167
  loss, 85
  muscle and, 162
  nutrition and, 133–135
wellness
  age reversal and, 16–21
  assessing, 28–33
  cell hydration and, 15–16, 18–21
  hydration and, 21–26
  Inclusive Health and, 26–28
  Phase Angle (PA) as measure of, 15–16, 19
  self-assessment, 28–33
  wellness water, 22–23, 40–41
  See also Inclusive Health care
whole fruit jam/spreads, 106–107
whole-wheat bread, 64
women
  alcohol consumption by, 167
  bone health of, 171
  facial hair and stress, 228–229
  fat *vs.* muscle, 169
  heart attacks in, 224
  menopause, 42–45, 49, 197–198
worry journals, 94
wrinkles, 184–185, 195–196

yoga, 175, 236
yogurt, 116

z-band filaments, 173
zinc, 72
zucchini, 64